Alkaline Diet for Beginners

The Unique Alkaline Foods Guide for Natural Weight Loss through a Plant Based Diet. Eat Well and Reclaim your Health for Unlimited Energy with a 21 Days Meal Plan

Marla Wilson

Table Of Contents

Introduction

Before we begin, I would like to thank you for purchasing this book, "Alkaline Diet for Beginners."

Over the years, our diets have evolved in a very different ways compared to how our ancestors ate. Unfortunately, most of the changes in our diet have been for the worse. They have had a negative impact on our well-being and consist mostly of unhealthy food that puts a strain on our metabolism and overall health. Thankfully, people have started paying attention to their health again and have become more conscious about the food they eat. If you are reading this book, you are probably one of them, as well. The best thing to do is find a holistic solution that will benefit you in more ways than one. This is where this book comes in.

If you have heard of this diet, you might have wondered what exactly it is. Maybe you know a little about it already--but just in case, we have put together enough information in this book for any beginner (or even expert) to benefit from it. The people who have followed this diet claim that it helps them lose weight, improve health and even fight various diseases. However, if you are still be feeling skeptical about all that, this book will help to clear all your doubts.

The basic concept is that the alkaline diet helps to restore the healthy pH balance of your body, which is necessary for optimum health. You will understand this in detail after reading through the various sections of this book. Unlike fad diets, you will not be asked to fast for days or survive on liquids or raw vegetables alone. There is no calorie counting required either. You already know that eating healthy food will help you stay healthy. On the other hand, unhealthy junk food will have a negative impact on your health. The alkaline diet will help you make better food choices that will ensure better health.

As you read on, you will learn about what the alkaline diet is, how it works, how you will benefit from it and how to implement the diet into your lifestyle. You will also be able to use the various recipes given here for all types of meals as you go alkaline. There is no way that the diet will leave you feeling hungry, unsatisfied or even bored. The healthy plan with delicious recipes will be simple and effective in helping to restore your body to a healthy state.

Chapter One: What Is The Alkaline Diet?

Before we delve into the details, it is important to understand the basics. Do you know what the alkaline diet is? This section will help you learn about the basic principles of the alkaline diet.

Firstly, the alkaline diet is based on the theory that alkaline foods should replace acid-forming foods to improve health and prevent diseases. This concept is elaborated on in this chapter, and it will help you understand what the diet is and why this acid-alkaline balance is important.

The alkaline diet is a healthy and holistic diet that will improve your overall health and well-being. The diet employs simple and effective principles that will help to improve your digestive health in many ways. It is important to try to maintain the natural state of your body and keep your digestive system healthy; however, the unhealthy modern diet prevents us from doing that. It is easy to see the negative symptoms of this unhealthy lifestyle.

- Think of your eating habits daily.
- Do you eat your meals on time?
- Do you chew your food well before swallowing?
- How often do you eat home-cooked meals compared to junk food or takeout?
- Do you experience bloating, gas or acid reflux often?
- Do your energy levels fluctuate all day, leaving you tired more often than not?

For most people, the answers to these questions will be in the affirmative, and that is not how it should be. When you have unhealthy eating habits, there will be repercussions in the form of negative symptoms. These signs are used by the body to display bad health and suffering. The reason behind most digestive issues, in particular, is excessive acid. The solution to this problem is the alkaline diet. This diet will help to recharge your body and reset your metabolic system. This will help to restore health and ensure that you will experience high levels of energy all day.

The alkaline diet has many benefits that you will experience as you begin following the guidelines given in this book. You will learn in detail about these benefits in another chapter of the book. The point is, the diet is effective regardless of your age, gender, and general health. As long as you don't have some specific disease that requires certain dietary restrictions, this diet is safe for just about everyone. Just in case, you should consult your physician to make sure the diet is appropriate for you. Once you get the go-ahead and begin following the diet, you will experience various benefits, ranging from weight loss to increased vitality and rejuvenation. Although the diet will help you lose weight, the alkaline diet is not focused on this aspect--it is not a weight loss-centric diet plan. The goal of this diet is more all-encompassing than that, and it is focused on improving your overall health and wellness by restoring balance to your body.

While following the modern diet, people tend to eat too many processed carbs, full-fat dairy products, refined sugar, etc. All of these food choices result in an acid bath in your body. This takes a toll on it and leads to various issues related to the digestive system, liver, kidneys, and other internal organs and systems. This kind of unhealthy diet has resulted in an increase in cases of renal disease, hypertension, digestive issues and other chronic illnesses in the long term. The human body requires maintenance of its delicate pH balance to remain healthy and well. The modern diet prevents this by disturbing the healthy pH levels that our bodies need for optimal health. The alkaline diet aims to rectify this error and restore good health.

About pH

Let's try to gain a better understanding of pH first. Technically, pH is used to measure the number of hydrogen ions in a solution. "pH" stands for the power of hydrogen. The "p" is an abbreviation of *potenz*, which is the German word for power. "H" is the symbol for hydrogen in the periodic table of the elements. The pH level determines the acidity or alkalinity of any water-soluble substances. When you use the pH scale, you can identify them as acidic, neutral or basic. The scale itself has a range of 0 to 14. When the pH is exactly a 7, it is considered neutral. When the pH is less than 7, it is acidic. The closer it is to zero, the more acidic it is. When the pH is greater than 7, it is alkaline. The closer it is to 14, the more alkaline it is. This pH scale is used in the human body as well.

The natural state of your body will have a regulated level of pH, which will eliminate any excess acid. The human body has to be a little alkaline to be in good health. Usually, the pH of your blood and other fluids should be between the pH range of 7.365 and 7.45; however, this balance is impacted by the diet and lifestyle of the individual. The pH value varies in the different parts of the body as well. Certain body parts will be more acidic or more alkaline. Your saliva will have a pH range of 6.8 to 7.4. The skin tends to be more acidic and is in the pH range of 4 and 6.5; however, the stomach is highly acidic because of the presence of hydrochloric acid, and the pH will vary between 2 and 3.5. The pH of your urine will be variable because it depends on the way your body is trying to restore any imbalances that may be present at any given time.

The modern diet, with all its unhealthy food, is more acidifying. While we have increased our consumption of these foods, we have decreased our consumption of foods that help to neutralize the acidity; therefore the balance is disturbed, and there is more acid than there should be. According to research[1], this pH imbalance has resulted in most of the illnesses and diseases that people chronically suffer from these days. Out of all other pH levels, the

[1] Kellum, J. A. (2000). Determinants of blood pH in health and disease. *Critical care (London, England)*, 4(1), 6–14. doi:10.1186/cc644

one of the highest significance in the human body is blood pH. This should always be in the range of 7.365 and 7.45. The numbers may appear simple for all these pH levels, but it is hard for the body to maintain these optimal numbers. When an acid needs to be neutralized, the body needs ten times the alkalinity for to be able to accomplish this. This means that the pH is operated on a scale of 10, and that the scale is exponential. So, jumping from one number to another on the pH scale may seem simple, but is a lot of work. If you compare the acidity level at pH 4 and pH 7, the acidity at pH 4 is a thousand times more than that at pH 7. You don't have to stress about these numbers too much, but it is important to have a basic understanding of how pH works if you want to understand the alkaline diet. Your body naturally knows what the healthy range of pH is, so the regulation will happen as long as you follow a healthy diet and lifestyle.

Therefore, we advocate the alkaline diet to counteract this. However, while alkalinity is important, it does not mean that you will not be consuming any acidic foods whatsoever. Certain foods, like lemons, will have an acidic pH, but their effect on the body after consumption serves to restore alkalinity. You have to understand that the pH level of the food itself is not enough to determine whether or not it is appropriate for the alkaline diet.

A lot of research has been conducted to understand how the body works. This is why it has been clear for a long time that the human diet affects the acid-base balance of the human body. When you eat certain foods, your body breaks them down. Energy is obtained from this breakdown, and the foods are digested in a slow, methodical way. The thing is, energy is not the only thing that is extracted from the breakdown of food. There are various other byproducts as well. These byproducts from your food may either be acidic, neutral or alkaline in nature. It will depend on what the food itself contained in terms of sulfur, protein or minerals. When the digested food has too much of an acidic byproduct left, it can cause inflammation in your body. This usually results from eating refined or processed foods, too many carbs, and sugars. This increase in inflammation makes your body vulnerable to illness and disease. The excessive acid may not be fatal by itself, but it can cause other diseases that, over time, just might become so. The body naturally tries to neutralize the burden of acids by using alkaline minerals. This helps to eliminate excess acid. In a healthy person, this feedback mechanism works effectively; however, when you follow a very unhealthy diet, the body is not able to function the same way. There will be too much acid and too little alkalizing constituents to neutralize or eliminate the excess acid effectively. This build-up of acid can have an extremely negative impact on your organs, organ systems, and your body as a whole. Excessive consumption of acid-producing food can wreak havoc on your body. It makes your body have to work even harder to try to normalize the pH, but the imbalance remains despite the body's efforts.

You should also know that your body is suffering not just because of your diet but due to other external factors as well. There is too much pollution, too many viruses, antibiotic-resistant bacterial strains, etc. these days and all of these add stress to your body too. The body will release stress hormones to combat against these physical stressors. These hormones include cortisol, insulin and adrenaline. Digestion is also slowed down to a sluggish, unhealthy pace. The food you ingest is not digested efficiently, and your digestive system suffers for it. The nutrients from food are not absorbed as they should be and this, in turn, causes more issues for your health. It is not uncommon for a modern person to have plenty of (albeit unhealthy) food to eat, yet suffer from malabsorption of nutrients and malnutrition as a result. When taking pH balance into consideration, it's no wonder why.

The alkaline diet will work to counteract the harmful impact of your unhealthy diet and strive to return your body to a healthy state. According to recent research[2] conducted in this field, it is recommended that consumption of plants be increased in the diet while ingestion of non-plant-based foods should be

---

[2] Katherine Marengo LDN, R. (2019). Alkaline diet: Claims, facts, and foods. Retrieved from
https://www.medicalnewstoday.com/articles/324271.php

reduced; therefore there are foods that you should and should not eat--both while you follow this diet and also in the long run. You will learn more about food choices and the diet plan later in the book.

Chapter Two: Guidelines For The Alkaline Diet

The alkaline diet is made up of various guidelines that will assist you with restoring balanced pH levels in your body by adjusting your intake of acidic or alkaline foods. It is important for people to pay attention to their diet over the years. Food is essential for health, and your diet should be comprised of foods that will benefit you and not harm you; however, the standard modern diet works in the opposite way and does more harm than good. As you follow the alkaline diet, you have to keep certain things in mind in order to make it to work effectively for you. Disregard any dietary myths you might have heard from your peers and aim to change the food habits that you have grown accustomed to. The principles shared in this chapter will help you rectify any bad eating habits and restore balance in terms of nutrition and lifestyle with the alkaline diet.

Practice Mindfulness

Most people these days tend to multitask while eating or rush through their meals. They like watching TV or reading a book while they absentmindedly eat. Or they might just grab a bite to eat when they can in their busy day. This means they barely pay attention to the food they are eating and don't even chew it well before swallowing. It is important to address this problem by practicing mindfulness. You need to be more aware of your body and what it is trying to tell you. Be more conscious of the dietary and lifestyle choices you are making. Think about it and you will see that a lot of the unconscious choices you have been making were detrimental to your health. Even the simplest thing, like washing down food with water, is a bad choice. However, you can change these choices, and make better decisions that can have a positive long-term impact on your health. Timely meals are a necessity for good health, but people compromise on it and take their health for granted. It is important for each person to set aside time for their meals and solely focus on the food they eat. Try to set aside 30 minutes for every main meal. Find a place to sit comfortably and be grateful for every good meal you receive. Don't be impatient when you eat; take time to enjoy your meal. Any work can be done later. Chewing food thoroughly is essential for good digestion. Take small bites and chew well before you swallow. Don't rush each bite and shove food down your throat. Eat your meal until you feel satisfied, but avoid overeating-- you want to feel full, but not stuffed. Your meal should be both nourishing and satiating.

Eat during meal times and don't fall prey to emotional eating. Don't eat when you are in a hurry or when you are stressed or upset. Your meal should be about nourishment; you cannot feed your feelings. This develops into an unhealthy habit that can lead to eating disorders. Be relaxed when you eat each meal so you can enjoy your nourishment to its fullest.

What You Eat Is Important

You should not eat everything just because it technically counts as food. Good food is different from unhealthy food that tastes good.

Your taste buds can be tricked into craving artificial flavors that overwhelm the palate and bog down the body with acidity. Acidic and alkaline foods need to be in balance in your diet. The amount of acidic food you eat should be half of the amount of alkaline foods you eat. Eat more whole foods and try to cut out minimally nutritious, questionable junk foods and processed foods. Beverages should also be alkalizing. You will learn more about alkaline foods and acidic foods in later chapters.

Constant Hydration

Hydration is important regardless of what diet you may choose to follow. Food is an important part of life, but so is water. They are both essential for survival; however, you need to drink a lot more water than you need to eat of food. The majority of people these days are chronically dehydrated. They don't drink even half of the amount of water that they are supposed to drink each day. This dehydration has a much bigger impact on their quality of life than they realize. Not drinking sufficient water can make you feel irritated, give you headaches, and make you feel lazy and tired all day long. When you start hydrating yourself properly, you will notice the difference it makes--and what a difference it is. Your health will improve, energy levels increase, and your immune system will be boosted. The quality of water matters too, so try to check that the pH level is between 8 to 9.5. Increasing hydration is easy and it has a huge impact on your health and how you feel.

First off, aim to drink at least six glasses of water in a day at minimum, and the number can go up to 18 glasses. The amount required for each person will depend on his or her body weight and activity level. One easy rule to determine this is drinking enough water to equal half your body weight measured in ounces. Add lemon water to your routine. You can take some lukewarm water and add juice from a freshly squeezed lemon into this. This lemon drink in the morning will help to flush toxins out your system and will ignite your metabolic system. It will buffer any excess acids and cleanse your digestive system. Another way to stay hydrated is to drink some herbal tea that will have additional benefits for your health. Use apps to remind you to take a water break once in a while. When the habit is built, your body will remind you that you missed that glass of water you sorely needed, without requiring any notifications from your phone.

Going Green Is Crucial For The Alkaline Diet

You have heard it time and again that green

foods are good for your health; however, most people don't pay heed to this and just eat as they please. The alkaline diet will guide you in adding more alkaline green foods back into your diet. Leafy greens, vegetables, and any fresh alkaline produce are all good for health.

Take Time For The Transition

There is no rush, nor is there any time limit when it comes to the alkaline diet. The current lifestyle you lead has been built over a period of many years. It will take time to transition from this lifestyle to a newer, healthier one; however, if you rush it and overwhelm yourself, it is not likely to be a successful transition. Instead, you will probably end up backsliding into eating the same junk food you previously consumed on a daily basis. If you try to follow the diet to the point right from the first day, you are setting yourself up for failure. This applies to any diet that you try for the first time. The alkaline diet is not restrictive so you can start by making conscious decisions to eat a little healthier from the first day. Instead of ordering takeout, try making something at home. Alternatively, order a healthy salad at a restaurant instead of cheesy pasta doused in copious amounts of white sauce. It is easy to know what is healthy and what is not, so you don't need to refer to the list given here all the time, either; however, you can use the alkaline and acidic food list provided later on in the book as a handy guide. Coming back to the main point, be mindful when eating your meals and just try to do a little better than you did yesterday. Trust the process. Slow progress is better than a fast failure.

Practice Breathing Exercises

Don't skip over this particular point. While you may be wondering what breathing has to do with diet, bear in mind that a healthy body requires certain healthy practices and good food alone will not do the trick. Practicing some simple breathing exercises each day can be immensely beneficial to your health, plus it helps you engage in more mindfulness. You can try to meditate for better effect, but breathing exercises themselves are simple and easy to practice. The increased oxygen flow from these exercises also helps to combat excess acid. Just find a comfortable place where you won't be disturbed. Sit and close your eyes. Breathe in, hold your breath and breathe out. Do the entire thing slowly and comfortably and repeat. Try to do this for ten reps to begin with, and do it regularly. It will help to clear your mind and help you focus better for the rest of the day too.

Opt For Alkaline Inducing Supplements

Many people are confused about what supplements they can have while following the alkaline diet. For one, you can try green powder, which is made from powdered wheatgrass, barley grass, fruit, vegetables, and sprouts. Also add alkaline mineral supplements like magnesium and potassium to up your electrolytes and help to buffer acids in your body. Alkaline water is a supplement that is made with pH drops, water ionizer, and some lemon juice. Omega oils are also a good supplement to consume as they have various benefits and are a healthy fat source.

The tips given here will help you as you start your transition to the alkaline diet. If you want to see real improvement, you need to make a real effort. Keeping these guidelines in mind as you begin your alkaline diet journey will help you make conscious healthy decisions about your diet and your habits in general.

Chapter Three: Impact Of An Acidic Diet

Let's take a look at the hazards of continuing on with an acidic diet. This will give you a better idea of how your current diet is harmful to your health.

Our ancestors followed a diet that had a good balance of acidic and alkaline foods; however, we have strayed too far from that diet in the modern era. The older diet was more wholesome and nutritious, and included an abundance of fruits, vegetables, nuts, and seeds. The present-day diet contains too much meat, too many grains, refined sugars, and other acid-inducing foods.

The result of following the present-day diet is that most of us have developed a condition called chronic low-grade metabolic acidosis. Your natural system has a feedback mechanism to handle occasional acid loads; however, when the amount of acid is excessive and builds up over time, the alkaline resources in your body are not sufficient to heal the damage done. The acids need to be neutralized, or else they cause imminent health damage. This acid-based diet is one of the main reasons that people of the modern generation are increasingly susceptible to diseases like osteoporosis.

Food should be eaten in moderation, and excess consumption should be avoided. When choosing which foods to eat, it is best to keep most of your diet plant-based. The problem in the modern diet is that it is too processed and most of the natural ingredients used in them lose their nutrients due to this overprocessing. If you study the content of most of the store-bought ingredients, they have surprising amounts of sodium, hidden sugars, and unhealthy fats. You don't have to cut all fat from your diet to lose weight. What is important is differentiating between healthy and unhealthy fats. In the present-day diet, there is too much of processed food along with animal proteins and these increase acidity. The acid levels are not balanced because of the lack of fruit and vegetable intake; therefore, the imbalanced ratio leads to poor health, illness and disease.

The food industries have replaced the potassium and magnesium in your food with high amounts of sodium. This is another factor that has led to potassium deficiency and too high of an acid load. The increased acid load has caused most people to be in a constant state of metabolic acidity. Another side effect is inflammation in various parts of your body. Acute inflammation is when your body is responding to something like a cut. This type of inflammation is necessary for good health and proper immune function. Chronic inflammation is when the process goes awry, and your health is undermined. The only good thing about this is that it can be reversed. Eating alkaline foods will restore the pH balance and reduce chronic inflammation. The human body requires a stable pH to work well; therefore, it reacts to the increased acid load by trying to restore balance. However, these attempts to restore balance just lead to more metabolic waste, muscle wasting and higher risk for developing chronic diseases. Studies[3] show that reduction of acid-producing foods will help to lower acid levels and reduce the strain on the natural buffering system of your body. It can thus help to delay or prevent various negative conditions, such as kidney stone formation. If you want a healthy and

---

3 Kresser, C. The Acid-Alkaline Myth: Part 1 (2019). Retrieved from https://chriskresser.com/the-ph-myth-part-1/

disease-free body, you need to neutralize the acid produced in your body with the alkaline diet.

PRAL

Have you heard about PRAL? It is an abbreviation for "Potential Renal Acid Load" of foods. Foods cannot be haphazardly categorized under acidic and alkaline. The PRAL of a food can be used to measure the level of acidity and alkalinity within it. On the PRAL scale, foods will have a score that is neutral, negative or positive. When the PRAL score is negative, the food is alkaline. Broccoli has a PRAL score of -1.2, so it is considered alkaline. When the PRAL score is positive, the food is acidic. Beef has a PRAL score of +7.8, so it is considered acidic. The score is determined depending on how many minerals, how much phosphorus and how much protein a food leaves behind after it is metabolized. Foods with a lot of protein or phosphorous will be acidic after metabolizing because they break down as sulfuric acid and phosphoric acid in the body. On the other hand, alkaline food residues will be trace minerals like magnesium and calcium, which are alkaline in nature.

Foods with a basic (alkaline) effect and negative value on the PRAL scale:

Fruits And Vegetables Under This Category

- Unsweetened apple juice
- Carrot juice
- Cocoa with skim milk
- Herbal tea
- Lemon juice
- Tomato juice
- Vegetable juice

- Dry white wine
- Coffee, infusion
- Grape juice
- Green tea
- Mineral water
- Unsweetened orange juice
- Red wine
- Espresso
- Beetroot juice
- Draft beer
- Margarine
- Hazelnuts
- Apples
- Apricots
- Bananas
- Figs
- Black currants
- Orange
- Pineapple
- Strawberries
- Watermelon

- Cherries
- Grapes
- Kiwi
- Lemon
- Apple cider vinegar
- Parsley
- Wine vinegar
- Brown sugar
- Honey
- Asparagus
- Broccoli
- Brussel sprouts
- Cauliflower
- Chicory
- Kale
- Kohlrabi
- Leek

Foods With A Neutral Value:

- Olive oil
- Sunflower seed oil

- Kefir cheese, full-fat
- White sugar

Foods With A Positive Value And Acidic Effect:

- Carp
- Cod
- Prawns
- Eel
- Salmon
- Trout
- Zander
- Sole
- Shrimps
- Pale beer
- Carbonated cola drinks (soda pop)
- Sardine
- Peanuts
- Walnuts

- Amaranth
- Barley
- Oat flakes
- Rye flour
- Wheat flour
- Rice
- Ox liver
- Pork
- Turkey
- Duck
- Lamb
- Veal
- Buttermilk
- Sausage
- Cottage cheese
- Yogurt
- Chicken
- Bread
- Rusk
- Salami

Signs Of An Acidic Diet:

- You will gain weight easily
- You will suffer from random pains in your muscles, bones or joints
- You will suffer from heartburn or acid reflux
- You might experience irritable bowel syndrome or intestinal cramping
- There will be a constant feeling of tiredness or fatigue
- Muscle loss or weakness
- You might suffer from receding gums
- Risk of developing kidney stones is higher
- There might be bone loss
- You will suffer from skin problems like acne
- Your skin and hair will be lackluster
- Higher risk of urinary tract problems

- Poor digestion in general

If you experience a few or more of these signs, your diet is too acidic. An acidic environment in your body is the perfect setting to harbor illness or disease.

Side Effects Of Acidic Foods

Let's take a look at the side effects of acidic foods in a little more detail.

Bone Density Is Lowered

Research[4] shows that acid-forming foods may cause an increase in calcium loss through urine. This leads to reduced bone density and can even lead to conditions such as osteoporosis and osteopenia. In a study conducted on this topic, a group of people was

---

[4] Frassetto, L., Banerjee, T., Powe, N., & Sebastian, A. (2018). Acid Balance, Dietary Acid Load, and Bone Effects-A Controversial Subject. *Nutrients*, *10*(4), 517. doi:10.3390/nu10040517

divided into two groups. Each group was given either acidic or an alkaline-based diet plan to follow. At the end of the study, the inference was that those who stuck to the acidic diet had an increase in calcium loss through urine by a significant percentage. Research[5] also shows that lower bone density is more likely in people who consume low amounts of calcium and consume more acidic foods.

Increased Acid Reflux

Acid reflux is gastroesophageal reflux disease (GERD). In this condition, the acid from the stomach tends to move back up the digestive tract and into the esophagus. This causes symptoms of acid reflux like chest pain or heartburn. In a healthy body, the esophagus will use its sphincter muscles to close and prevent the backflow of stomach

---

[5] Sunyecz, J. A. (2008). The use of calcium and vitamin D in the management of osteoporosis. *Therapeutics and clinical risk management*, 4(4), 827–836.

acid so it remains within the stomach where it belongs; however, the acidic diet causes GERD, which weakens or damages the sphincter muscles and prevents efficient functioning. Foods like caffeinated drinks or high-fat food can be common triggers for this condition. The symptoms can be reduced with the help of following an alkaline diet.

Kidney Stone Formation

The pH of urine is affected by the foods that you eat. More acidic food will cause the urine pH to be acidic as well. The acidic pH, in turn, increases the chances of a person developing kidney stones. These are small mineral depositions from the food you eat, and they form like stones in the kidney. They can be (painfully) passed through the urinary tract but might even have to be removed surgically or broken down via sounding before they can pass. Avoid foods that are rich in oxalates, sodium and animal protein to prevent kidney stone formation.

Hormonal Levels Are Altered

The European Journal of Nutrition University of California published research that came out of the University of California[6] that showed how acidosis might decrease human growth hormone levels. This hormone is secreted by the pituitary gland in the body and is essential for growth and cell regeneration. Another study conducted on children with familial renal tubular acidosis showed that an alkaline diet helped in the elevation of their growth rate over time.

These are just some of the negative effects that a highly acidic diet has on your body. You can learn more about this in the section

---

[6] Schwalfenberg, G. K. (2011). The alkaline diet: is there evidence that an alkaline pH diet benefits health? *Journal of environmental and public health, 2012,* 727630. doi:10.1155/2012/727630

related to the benefits of the alkaline diet.

Acid Reflux

Let us look at the signs of acid reflux in people, as this is a common occurrence for those who follow the present-day diet. For the vast majority of people with indigestion or acid reflux, manifestations include:

- Pain in the chest and a burning sensation
- Bitter taste on the tongue
- Trouble in resting well, including waking up with the feeling of gagging or coughing at night.
- Dry mouth
- Irritation in the gums and gums feeling tender or bleeding
- Awful breath
- Suffering from burping, gas or bloating after meals.

- Occasional queasiness and loss of hunger

What's more, there are a huge number of different side effects depending on how seriously the esophagus of the person is inflamed or damaged.

GERD indications are like indigestion symptoms, albeit at times progressively extreme. The fundamental reason that indigestion/acid reflux occurs is because of dysfunction of the lower esophageal sphincter (LES). Typically the LES "keeps a cover on things" by keeping acid from streaming back up through the throat. While the stomach has an internal coating that shields it from acidity, the throat does not. Since it's not protected like the stomach is, the throat can begin to disintegrate and create difficulties and pain after some time when indigestion isn't dealt with. Accordingly, tissue scarring and even esophageal malignant growths can occur in extreme cases.

Are All Acidic Foods Bad?

Not every single acidic food ought to be wiped out from the dietary routine. Some of these acidic foods give us significant supplements and can be incorporated into balance as a major aspect of a healthy dietary regimen. Most kinds of meat, for instance, are viewed as acidic yet supply many important nutrients and minerals to the body and can likewise enable you to meet your everyday protein needs to improve the well-being of your cells and muscles. Walnuts are also viewed as acidic sustenance, however they are wealthy in cancer prevention agents and omega-3 unsaturated fats, which can diminish irritation and advance better well-being. The key is to incorporate these acidic nourishments as a component of a solid, holistic, entire-sustenance diet and blend these healthy acidic foods with a lot of organic products, vegetables, and plant-based proteins also.

Tips for replacing unhealthy acidic foods with alkaline foods:

Following a low-corrosive eating regimen can be as straightforward as making a couple of basic substitutes and exchanging out sustenance that causes irritation for foods that advance better well-being. Here are a couple of thoughts for simple trades you can make to decrease acidic nourishments manifestations:

- Swap out your soda pops for basic water, and begin your day with a refreshing green smoothie rather than an espresso.
- Have a go at including a plant-based

protein, for example, beans or vegetables, in your dinner instead of meat a couple of times each week.

- Improve up your sugar habit by using raw sugars like crude nectar or maple syrup rather than refined sugars.

- Reduce the intake of highly processed foods and center your diet around natural sources of nourishment.

- Pick natural, fresh produce whenever possible, and search for grass-fed, unfenced or wild beef, poultry and fish.

Not every acidic food ought to be avoided totally. Indeed, a number of these acidic foods contain a great array of nutrients and can be a part of a solid dietary routine. Seeking out a balanced, adjusted eating regimen is the key, and you should concentrate on including antacid foods like natural products as opposed to restricting acidic foods like meats. Rather than fastidiously restricting or maintaining a limit on specific food groups, focus on filling your eating regimen with mostly natural, whole nutrients and you'll gain ground toward improved well-being.

Chapter Four: Negative Impact Of Animal Protein

Most proteins obtained from plants and animals are "complete proteins" (which means they contain the majority of the important amino acids we need); however, people use the expression "low quality" for plant proteins since they commonly have low levels of basic amino acids when compared with animal proteins. It's important to understand that having a higher amount of amino acids is actually harmful and can have a negative effect on our well-being.

Unlike like plant protein, which comes bundled with fiber, cell reformation, and phytonutrients, animal protein has none of the above. Eggs, meat, poultry, fish, dairy, and other animal products have no fiber at all. Numerous individuals, in their bid to "get enough" protein, eat a lot of animal protein, while avoiding plant proteins that contain all these significant supplements. Fiber insufficiencies, specifically, are undeniably more common than not. For instance, The Institute of Medicine suggests that men consume 38 grams of fiber, yet the average grown-up eats only around 15 grams each day—not exactly a large portion of the suggested amount. As indicated by the USDA, practically all Americans[7] (95%) don't get a satisfactory amount of dietary fiber. High fiber intake is related to lower malignancy risks, especially for colon and breast tumors, and can also lower danger of ulcerative colitis, Crohn's, intestinal blockages, and diverticulitis. It might likewise lessen the danger of stroke, high cholesterol, and heart disease.

---

[7] Quagliani, D., & Felt-Gunderson, P. (2016). Closing America's Fiber Intake Gap: Communication Strategies From a Food and Fiber Summit. *American journal of lifestyle medicine, 11*(1), 80–85. doi:10.1177/1559827615588079

When we consume proteins that have higher amounts of important amino acids (which is usually the case with animal protein), it results in our bodies delivering higher amounts of the hormone insulin-like growth factor-1 (IGF-1). This hormone strengthens cell division and development of both healthy and disease cells and, therefore, having higher flowing dimensions of IGF-1 has been reliably connected with the threat or cancerous growths.

Excess animal protein consumption results in us consuming higher amounts of trimethylamine N-oxide (TMAO). TMAO is a substance affects our blood vessels, causes irritation, and encourages the buildup of cholesterol plaques in our veins. What's more, it is exceptionally risky for cardiovascular health. TMAO is made by complex formations including our gut flora and the supplements in the proteins we eat. Furthermore, when we eat animal protein, it modifies our gut flora and encourages the formation of TMAO. In this way, excess consumption of animal protein can result in higher TMAO levels, which can be harmful to our body.

Animal protein contains large amounts of phosphorus. What's more, when we devour large quantities of phosphorus, one manner in which our bodies attempt to cope with the amount of phosphorus is with a hormone called Fibroblast Growth Factor 23 (FGF23). FGF23 can be destructive for our veins and other blood vessels. It can likewise prompt hypertrophy of the cardiovascular ventricle (irregular expansion of our heart muscle) and is related to heart attacks and heart failure, which can lead to untimely death. So eating animal protein with its high levels of phosphorus can result in an increase of this hormone in our bodies, which can be exceedingly hazardous for our well-being.

Iron is the most important metal in the human body. We can divide it in two types:

- Heme iron, usually found in animal proteins like meat, poultry, and fish;
- Non-heme iron, generally found in plants.

One of the issues with heme iron is that it can change less receptive oxidants into exceptionally responsive free radicals, and free radicals can harm all kinds of cell structures like proteins, films, and even the DNA. Heme iron can also catalyze the development of N-nitroso mixes in our bodies, which are strong cancer-causing agents. In this way, of course, high admission of heme iron has been related with numerous kinds of gastrointestinal problems and other pathologies.

The facts confirm that heme iron has higher ingestion rates and bioavailability than non-heme iron. Be that as it may, iron itself can cause oxidative pressure and DNA harm, so with iron, for the most part, it's not generally a circumstance where "more is better." While we certainly do need iron to survive (lest we become anemic due to insufficient blood iron), the assimilation and bioavailability of iron from a balanced, plant-based eating routine are typically completely satisfactory, and we can avoid the issues related with heme iron along with other negative properties of animal foods.

Animal proteins also have, all in all, higher groupings of sulfur-containing amino acids, which can prompt acidosis when they become metabolized. One of the systems our bodies use to make up for this acidosis is the process of draining calcium from our tissues. After some time, this can have a very negative impact on bone health. This is believed to be one reason why a few studies have led to the discovery that people with higher dairy intake, with higher utilization of animal protein when all is said and done, likewise have a higher frequency of bone fractures.

Most animal protein sources contain fat and cholesterol (this is valid for even purportedly "lean" meats like chicken, turkey, and salmon, paying little mind to how they are cooked or arranged—regardless of whether boiled, baked, fried or steamed). As humans, we don't have to consume any cholesterol, since our bodies produce all the cholesterol we require for our physiological needs. Consuming cholesterol regardless of this reality is risky for our well-being, as it increases the danger of developing coronary illness, which is presently the number 1 reason for death for people in the United States. Atherosclerosis, or plaques of cholesterol that collect in the covering of our blood vessels, is less common when on a plant-based veggie-heavy diet without animal foods.

Chapter Five: Benefits Of The Alkaline Diet

If you need more information to be convinced about the benefits of the alkaline diet, look no further. This section of the book is solely focused on summarizing all the benefits that you can reap by making the change to an alkaline diet.

Aids In Weight Loss

Many people try the alkaline diet to help in weight loss. One of the simplest ways the diet helps is that it suggests replacing unhealthy, non-nutritious and acid-inducing foods with healthy, alkalinizing substitutes that are low in calories. The foods in the alkaline diet are richer in nutrients, and they support gut health while boosting the immune system. This helps to burn calories and maintain a healthy weight.

Reduced Risk Of Hypertension, Strokes Or Heart Disease

Various studies[8] have been conducted on adults with high blood pressure. More than 30% of adults in the current generation suffer from high blood pressure. This increases their risk of strokes and heart disease. One of the main causes of these conditions is following an unhealthy diet. The risk of high blood pressure is directly linked to the human diet. The modern-day diet does not contain sufficient

---

[8] Drozdz, D., & Kawecka-Jaszcz, K. (2013). Cardiovascular changes during chronic hypertensive states. *Pediatric nephrology (Berlin, Germany)*, 29(9), 1507–1516. doi:10.1007/s00467-013-2614-5

amounts of healthy vegetables and fruits, but instead involves excessive consumption of animal products. This results in metabolic acidosis and the pH of urine becomes reduced. These high acid levels will increase the likelihood of the person suffering from hypertension and heart disease related to it. The alkaline diet comes to the rescue by adding a high amount of potassium and magnesium into your diet and these, in turn, will promote healthy blood pressure levels. The mineral ratio is shifted to a more positive range, and the risk of heart disease is reduced when you follow the alkaline diet.

Improvement In Digestive Health

Digestive health is largely determined by diet. When you consume massive amounts of animal protein, it has a negative effect on your gut over time; however, alkaline-rich foods will help to reduce the risk of many metabolic and inflammatory conditions. Studies[9] show that the alkaline-friendly Mediterranean diet helps to protect people from Crohn's disease. Alkaline foods, in general, are better alternatives as staples in the diet to help you battle any digestive distress or illness.

Reduces The Risk Of Kidney Stone Formation

Recent studies[10] show that one in every eleven people in the USA is at risk for developing kidney stones at some point in their lifetime. The modern diet is high in sodium, sugar and animal protein, which

[9] Saxena, A., Kaur, K., Hegde, S., Kalekhan, F. M., Baliga, M. S., & Fayad, R. (2014). Dietary agents and phytochemicals in the prevention and treatment of experimental ulcerative colitis. *Journal of traditional and complementary medicine, 4*(4), 203–217. doi:10.4103/2225-4110.139111

[10] Alelign, T., & Petros, B. (2018). Kidney Stone Disease: An Update on Current Concepts. *Advances in urology, 2018*, 3068365. doi:10.1155/2018/3068365

promote the formation of kidney stones. These nutrients are too excessive for the kidneys to filter efficiently and therefore, they remain within the kidneys and congeal together into kidney stones. A high-sodium diet, in particular, is a cause for concern as calcium levels become significantly increased. These stone-promoting nutrients like sodium and phosphorus can lead to low-grade metabolic acidosis. This is a bigger problem for older people as compared with those who are younger. Younger people can filter these nutrients more easily, but kidney function tends to decrease in efficiency with advanced age. One of the best predictors of kidney stone formation is a high amount of dietary acids. When you start the alkaline diet, it will help to reduce the load of stone-promoting nutrients.

Immune System Boost

The alkaline diet will increase your intake of antioxidants and reduce the toxins in your body so the immune system can focus on fighting off any illness. Diets that call for an increase in the intake of fresh vegetables and fruit can help people by strengthening their immunity. People following these types of diets are much less likely to fall ill compared to those who don't.

Prevents The Loss Of Muscle Mass

The human body tends to lose muscle mass as it ages. Apart from the passage of time, another contributing factor is an inactive lifestyle and an unhealthy diet. Loss of muscle mass will prevent effective burning of calories in the body, and this is why many people tend to gain weight as they grow older. Lower muscle mass will also make you more susceptible to falls and injuries that can affect your ability to move around independently. According to a study that was published in the *American Journal of Clinical Nutrition*, consuming an alkaline-rich diet will reduce acid load and thus preserve muscle mass as you age. Just adding a little more alkaline foods to balance out your pH levels can help to ensure healthy body movements over time.

Prevention Of Type 2 Diabetes

Type 2 diabetes cases have increased over the years, and the rates are higher now than in any other prior generation. This disease can be prevented to a large extent if the right precautionary measures are taken. According to one study[11], one of the steps you can take

---

[11] Han, E., Kim, G., Hong, N., Lee, Y. H., Kim, D. W., Shin, H. J., ... Cha, B. S. (2016). Association between dietary acid load and the risk of

is reducing the dietary acid load in your body because it increases the risk of diabetes when acid levels are too high. Studies[12] link high dietary acid levels directly to a higher risk of type 2 diabetes. If you increase alkaline food consumption and try to maintain a healthy body weight, this disease can be prevented, or at the very least, the risk of developing it is significantly lowered.

Reduced Risk Of Cancer

No firm clinical proof confirms the correlation between acid and cancer; however, diet-induced acidosis has the potential of increasing the risk of cancer. Some studies[13]

cardiovascular disease: nationwide surveys (KNHANES 2008-2011). *Cardiovascular diabetology*, *15*(1), 122. doi:10.1186/s12933-016-0436-z

[12] White, D. L., & Collinson, A. (2013). Red meat, dietary heme iron, and risk of type 2 diabetes: the involvement of advanced lipoxidation end products. *Advances in nutrition (Bethesda, Md.)*, *4*(4), 403–411. doi:10.3945/an.113.003681

[13] Schwalfenberg G. K. (2011). The alkaline diet: is there evidence that an alkaline pH diet benefits health?. *Journal of environmental and public health*, *2012*, 727630. doi:10.1155/2012/727630

show that an alkaline diet can help to manipulate urine pH levels so that chemotherapy is more effective on cancer patients. Certain dieticians also suggest an alkaline diet when a person undergoes chemotherapy. The alkaline diet itself is very similar to the diet that is suggested in general for people undergoing cancer treatment. It is recommended that these persons increase the consumption of fruits and vegetables daily while they reduce consumption of any processed or red meat, sodium, and alcohol.

Treatment Of Chronic Lower Back Pain

Certain studies[14] suggest that alkaline minerals can be beneficial for those suffering

---

[14] Sedighi, M., & Haghnegahdar, A. (2014). Role of vitamin D3 in treatment of lumbar disc herniation--pain and sensory aspects: study protocol for a randomized controlled trial. *Trials, 15,* 373. doi:10.1186/1745-6215-15-373

from a case of chronic lower back pain. Increasing magnesium consumption in particular can help improve the functioning of enzyme systems and help with the activation of vitamin D. Both of these can help to reduce pain in the lower back. The bottom line is that an alkaline diet will help to improve or ease the symptoms associated with chronic lower back pain.

You can see that consuming an alkaline diet, which is rich in fresh produce, will benefit your health much more than any other diet plan. It will help to prevent as well as promote healing from various illnesses. You will find it much easier to attain your weight loss goals healthily and efficiently, while enjoying all the other benefits of reducing bodily acid load at the same time. The alkaline diet is one of the best ways to ensure good gut health and overall well-being.

Overview of the benefits of the alkaline diet:

- Improvement in digestion
- Reduced bloating
- Youthful and clear skin by the elimination of acne
- Restful sleep.
- Abundance of energy
- Diminished fatigue
- Reduced pains or aches caused by gout, arthritis or headaches
- Immunity boost that protects you from frequent colds or other viral infections
- Increase in mental clarity and improved ability to remain alert
- Improvement in mental well-being-- Mood remains uplifted, and you feel happier
- Reduced risk of osteoporosis development caused due to acidity

- Reduced risk of cancer and improvement in chemotherapy effects
- Reversal or prevention of many chronic conditions

All of these are the effects that other alkaline diet followers have claimed to experience after changing their way of eating. You may benefit from these too if you follow the same healthy alkaline diet for yourself.

Chapter Six: Foods to Avoid on The Alkaline Diet

It is not always so easy to identify what is alkaline and what is not. This section of the book will help you learn about the foods you need to avoid or control when you begin the alkaline diet. The next section will help you learn about the foods that you should increase consumption of while on the alkaline diet. So, let's get started with outlining the foods to avoid.

You now know that foods cannot be identified as acidic or alkaline based on their taste or appearance. Many people consider a lemon acidic, but it is alkalinizing. You might be wondering how this is possible since it tastes so tart. Well, the lemon is acidic by nature but has an alkalizing effect when it is metabolized in the body; therefore, it is an alkaline forming food that you don't have to avoid. Similarly, you need to identify foods that turn acidic after they are metabolized by the body and avoid these. The acidic nature of a food does not mean they will form acid in your body after being metabolized. Sauerkraut is an acidic food, but it will be alkalizing in your body. The PRAL scale mentioned in a previous section of the book is a more accurate way to measure the acidity and alkalinity of foods. This is what is used for determining what you should avoid on the alkaline diet. Anything with a positive PRAL food is acidic and should be avoided or else consumed less of. When you check the PRAL index of your current diet, you will understand what we are talking about.

- Fish and seafood have a positive value on the PRAL table and are acidic in effect. Avoid or limit consumption of carp, herring, salmon, prawns, sardines, trout, zander, tiger prawns, sole, shrimp, rosefish, haddock, halibut, eel, and cod.

- Beverages like pale beer are also acidic. Avoid sugary drinks and sodas like Coca-Cola. Any juices you drink should be from natural ingredients and without sweeteners.

- Avoid unhealthy fat sources like salted butter.

- Nuts to avoid include pistachio, peanuts, and sweet almonds.

- Cereals and flours are a major acidic contributor. Avoid consumption of white rice, wheat flour, oat flakes, corn flakes, corn, unripe spelt grains, and rye flour. Also avoid macaroni, spaghetti, and similar noodles.

- Avoid bread or limit how often you consume it. This includes bread made from rye flour, wheat flour, coarse wholemeal, pumpernickel, rusk, and white wheat. Bread adds a lot of carbs and causes weight gain too.

- Reduce or avoid milk and dairy products. This includes buttermilk, sour cream, eggs, curd cheese, cottage cheese, cheddar cheese, Edam cheese, gouda, hard cheese, kefir cheese, whole milk, camembert, yogurt, skim milk, and full-fat cheese.

- Animal meat is excessively consumed in the modern diet. Avoid eating meat more than three times a week at the most. The meats to avoid include beef, chicken, veal, sausages, pork, liver from ox or pig, lean goose, lamb, lean duck, lean rabbit, rump steak, turkey and salami.

- Acidic sweets include bitter chocolate, milk chocolate, and dairy ice cream.

In general, you need to avoid the above-mentioned grains, sugar, dairy products, fish, fresh or processed meats, sodas, sweetened beverages, high-protein foods and just any highly processed foods or junk foods.

Chapter Seven: Foods Approved On The Alkaline Diet

Now that you know what not to eat, let's look at what you should eat more of. These are foods that are negative on the PRAL list and are alkaline forming in your body. In general, as you look at the list, you will see that it consists of wholesome, nutritious food guidelines that you learned about in school but did not follow. It is time to change that and to stabilize the pH level in your body for better health again.

Eat More Vegetables

You can should add a variety of vegetables to your diet like asparagus, basil, beetroot, broad beans, carrot, cabbage, broccoli,

Brussels sprouts, celery, chilis, coriander, cucumber, chard, chives, zucchini, endive, dandelion, cauliflower, eggplant, garlic, ginger, green beans, kale, kelp, lettuce, mint, new potato, onion, collards, parsley, peas, pumpkin, snow peas, string beans, sweet potato, wakame, watercress, radish, spinach, squashes, fennel, leeks, peppers, gherkin, rucola, sauerkraut, tomato and chicory.

Grains

Eat more of the grains and beans that are alkaline forming. These include amaranth, buckwheat, millet, quinoa, runner beans, millet, lima beans, lentils, kamut, chia, pinto beans, and mung beans.

Nuts And Seeds

Nuts and seeds are a great addition to the

alkaline diet. Add almonds, coconut, flax seeds, sunflower seeds, hazelnuts, pumpkin seeds and sesame seeds for alkaline effect.

Grasses

You can also add alkaline grasses to your diet like wheatgrass, shave grass, oat grass, dog grass, barley grass, and kamut grass.

Fruits

Fruits are my personal favorite part of the diet. There are so many to choose from so try any of the fruits mentioned here. Alkaline forming fruits include apples, bananas, apricots, grapefruit, grapes, orange, raisins, strawberries, mango, peach, watermelon, lemon, orange, cherries, kiwi, figs, papaya, black currants, avocado, and coconut.

Bread

Alkaline bread includes sprouted bread, sprouted wraps, and gluten- or yeast-free breads are your best bet while on an alkaline diet.

Vinegar

Apple cider vinegar and wine vinegar are alkaline-forming types and recommended on the diet.

Oil

The alkaline diet recommends using avocado oil, coconut oil, flaxseed oil, olive oil, and Udo's oil.

Beverages

Beverages should have a negative value on the PRAL list. These include unsweetened apple juice, beetroot juice, herbal tea, unsweetened orange juice, dry white wine, red wine, vegetable juice, grape juice, lemon juice, mineral water, espresso, fruit tea, stout beer, draft beer, and infusion coffee.

Dessert

If you are someone who loves dessert, stick to brown sugar, marmalade, honey, and nougat hazelnut cream.

If the foods are mentioned in this book, you can go ahead and consume them while following the guidelines of the alkaline diet. None of these are acid forming and will help to neutralize excess acids in your body. You can try the delicious recipes outlined later in this book as you use these ingredients to push your body back to a healthy state.

Alkaline Water

I am adding a section on alkaline water because it is a common part of alkaline diets. If you have read about or talked of the alkaline diet, the chances are that alkaline water came up at some point.

Alkaline water is the opposite of acidic water. Experts suggest that you try to drink water that is less acidic than the regular tap water that most people drink.

So, what is alkaline water? Alkaline water is water that is rich in compounds that have an alkalizing effect. These alkaline compounds include calcium, magnesium, bicarbonate, potassium, and silica. The pH of this alkaline water will be between 8 and 9. Normal water has a neutral pH of 7. This pH level is affected by any chemicals or gases that the water is subjected to. They will determine how acidic or alkaline the water becomes. If you consider rainwater, the pH is a little less than 7, so it is acidic because of the carbon dioxide mixed in water from the air. It is okay for water to have a little high or low pH value, but the values should not be drastically different from the neutral pH level. If water is too alkaline, the taste will be bitter, and it can cause encrusting deposits in pipes or appliances. If the water is too acidic, it can cause corrosion of metals and even dissolve the metal. Alkaline water is water that is just a little less acidic than the regular tap water you have been drinking. The people who promote alkaline water claim that it can help to neutralize acid present in your bloodstream and also metabolize nutrients effectively. The proponents of this beverage believe that it will improve health and performance if consumed regularly.

However, I advise against paying too much attention to these claims and limiting alkaline water intake, if it is going to be consumed at all. It is too simple to say that this water will alkalize your body when the body is such a complex thing. The fact is that every organ system in your body has its unique range of pH levels. This pH level in different parts will also be affected for different reasons at times. Drinking alkaline water will not get rid of all the possible underlying causes. Knowing the real cause may help you decide if alkaline water really will help.

Potential Benefits Of Alkaline Water

A particular group of people who might benefit from drinking some alkaline water is people who exercise a lot or who are athletes. This alkaline water will help them to retain more fluid in their cardiovascular system than is needed for people with less active lifestyles. Their urine output will be reduced along with blood osmolality. The latter is linked to an elevated risk of fatal strokes in people, so this alkaline water is helpful; however, these beneficial effects in this group will not be instantly apparent. If they follow a plan and consume alkaline water over time, the gradual improvements will be visible, therefore, you can take into consideration that active people will benefit from regular hydration with normal water along with some alkaline water; however, there is no concrete evidence to prove this.

Better Hydration

When it comes to alkaline water benefits, there is something else to consider. Since you will be drinking more water, regardless of alkalinity or neutrality, you will notice some obvious improvement in health. These will be simply from the fact that hydration is increased even while you consume a processed modern diet. The change and effect will not make much of a difference for those who already follow a healthy alkaline or balanced diet and exercise regularly; however, active people will benefit due to other reasons that are less obvious and have nothing to do with hydration. When a person exercises intensely, their muscles will produce increased amounts of hydrogen ions. These are more than the amount the human body can efficiently get rid of by itself. This causes increased fatigue. In this case, alkaline water may help to enhance the buffering capacity of the body and will temper the acidity. This, in turn, will improve the performance of the person.

Prevention Of Toxins

Alkaline water can also protect you from certain toxins present in tap water. Tap water is regularly disinfected before it reaches your home. This is done to protect you from the bacteria or toxins that may be present in the water; however, the disinfectants used for this may react with organic matter and cause harmful byproducts. Disinfectant byproducts can cause a variety of health issues and are harmful to the environment, as well. This makes it a good reason to consider the fact that alkaline water breaks a few of these disinfectants' byproducts down and neutralizes their possible effect on us or the environment. This only applies to some byproducts because there are others that actually thrive in alkaline water. Nonetheless, the alkaline urine resulting from drinking alkaline water can also help in the removal of toxins from the body.

Gut Health May Benefit From Alkaline Water

There is something known as ORP or oxidation-reduction potential. It is the measure of a solution's tendency to gain or lose electrons when being subjected to change caused by the introduction of any new species. According to research[15], ORP has some effect on bacteria present in the gut. Ionized alkaline water possesses a negative ORP, therefore it may offer some disinfectant effect and protect you from the dangerous microorganisms that may be present in the water.

Prevents Liver Damage And Diabetes

If simple molecules of a sugar like fructose are attached to lipid fats or proteins without any enzyme moderation, a reaction called

---

[15] Circu, M. L., & Aw, T. Y. (2011). Redox biology of the intestine. *Free radical research*, 45(11-12), 1245–1266. doi:10.3109/10715762.2011.611509

"glycation" takes place. This reaction causes rogue molecule formation, and these are known as AGEs or "advanced glycation end products." Studies[16] link AGEs with a higher risk of Alzheimer's disease and diabetes. Drinking ionized alkaline water has the potential to lower glycation levels as well as reduce damage in the liver. These observations are obtained by the results seen while studying the effect of alkaline water on rats with blood pressure issues; therefore you need to keep this in mind and not attempt to generalize the data to humans. There is no tangible proof of the same effects being displayed in human beings.

These days, you can easily buy packaged alkaline water at grocery stores or drug stores. These products have become increasingly

---

[16] Lovestone, S., & Smith, U. (2014). Advanced glycation end products, dementia, and diabetes. *Proceedings of the National Academy of Sciences of the United States of America, 111*(13), 4743–4744. doi:10.1073/pnas.1402277111

popular among the new-age health fanatics that are trying out new health fads all the time. But you don't need to buy the fancy packaged water labeled as alkaline. Bottled mineral water is usually alkaline by nature. Bottled water that is not mineral-infused is less likely to be alkaline. You can add mineral powders to your regular tap water as a cheaper solution to create alkaline water yourself. If the water is very acidic, you will need to buy a water ionizer to create alkaline water. The tap water will undergo ionization in this machine and provide you with alkaline water; however, according to the majority of chemists, there is no meaning behind the term "ionized water," and they advise against buying ionizing machines. There are some who advocate on the contrary. The choice is ultimately yours to make. You can even look up the pH and ORP of the bottled waters that you purchase to find out about their alkalinity.

Although there is no hard evidence regarding the benefits of alkaline water, you can still try to add some to your diet when you begin. A limited amount of it will not cause any health issues, so you have nothing to lose by giving it a try and deciding for yourself whether it is a worthwhile addition to your diet. The diet itself, however, will do most of the work when it comes to reducing bodily acid load.

People who suffer from any kidney disease or dysfunction should avoid drinking alkaline water regularly. The alkaline minerals may accumulate in the kidneys of such people and escalate problems. Even if you don't have any imminent kidney issues, try to limit the amount of alkaline water you drink. Just because it can be helpful does not mean that more will work better. Normal mineral water will help you stay healthy and hydrated just the same.

Chapter Eight: Sample Alkaline Diet Plan

Creating An Alkaline Diet Plan

Now, let's get to it! It would help if you started on your alkaline diet plan as soon as you're done reading through this book. Delaying it will only allow your present dietary choices to harm your body further. The potential benefits of this diet have already been outlined to you, and there may even be more than those we have already covered. You won't know until you try it for yourself. Creating a plan for yourself will help you follow through with it. Once you stick to the plan for a few days, you will get the hang of it. The alkaline diet plan I give you in this section is just a simple guide to help you get started. You can make any adjustments according to what is convenient for you. There are so many wholesome ingredients that you can use, so there is no way that the diet gets boring or bland at any point. You can experiment with various recipes to make them more fun and better suited to your specific tastes. The only thing we recommend is to follow the lists given here as a guide.

You don't have to go head-on and make things hard for yourself. Take some baby steps, and you will find it easy soon enough. The diet is not complicated, nor is it demanding on anyone. You don't have to count calories, sacrifice meals for smoothies, fast or exercise multiples times in a day for it to be effective. The alkaline diet plan will help you to make the right dietary choices and avoid those foods that do more harm than good.

Before you begin, you have to take stock of

the food in the pantry and your house. Throw out junk food or any highly processed food that is highly acidic. Thankfully, the alkaline diet does not require you to get rid of everything you already have. You have to adjust the foods in a way that 80% of the food is alkaline and 20% can be acidic. So, keep this rule in mind when you start stocking up on groceries. There should be a lot of fresh produce with all the ingredients mentioned in the alkaline food list. These should fill up most of your cart while you can add a little portion of meat, dairy or anything else that is acidic.

The successful switching of diets is not as easy as some make it out to be. To prepare any of the alkaline recipes we suggest, you need to ensure that you have the ingredients required. You also need to invest the time required to prepare these meals. This is an essential part of the process, and you need to stop eating out as often as you currently do. A home-cooked meal allows you to remain in control of your diet to a greater extent because you know exactly what ingredients went into your meal. This control is lost when you try to grab quick meals at a deli or drive-through restaurant without any thought of what you are going to eat. You can still eat out, but always keep the ingredient list in mind. Choose foods on the menu that use ingredients that are alkaline. But in general, try to prepare your own meals with fresh ingredients. This is a lifestyle change that you will never regret in the long run. You can keep some lunches pre-packed and ready to go in the fridge to save you time too.

A meal plan is the best way to prepare yourself and stay on track with the alkaline diet. The recipes given in this book will help you enjoy the process. The food choices in the sample plan are simple, yet delicious too. These don't require any complicated cooking, and you can just toss them together. Adjust the amounts of each ingredient according to your personal choice. The plan does not contain many high-acid-forming foods, but you can add a little of these over time.

Use basic ingredients to make solid snacks and meals. Since greens are among the most antacid veggies, appreciating a major green serving of mixed greens on the soluble eating regimen is an easy decision.

On the off chance that you need an accommodating breakdown of what you ought to eat throughout the day, here's an example of an alkaline-eating routine menu. I will now give you a seven-day alkaline diet plan that will help you begin the process.

Day 1 Plan

Breakfast

Strawberry, quinoa, coconut, chia seeds with almond milk:

Cook the quinoa the previous night and get the strawberry chia ready by mixing the strawberries, almond milk, and two dates in a blender and pureeing it together until smooth. Empty the blend into a container and include chia seeds. Blend well until all chia seeds are held with the fluid. Keep it covered and refrigerate for the night. At the beginning of the next day, place chia seeds in a bowl, include the quinoa and strawberry cuts, almonds, and shaved coconut and appreciate the goodness of this healthy recipe!

Lunch

A sweet and savory salad with butter lettuce, cucumber, avocado, pomegranate, and extra virgin olive oil:

Just tear the lettuce into a plate of mixed greens. Include the remainder of the fixings and prepare with the dressing.

Dinner

Tofu stir fry with your choice of vegetables:

You can cut up any alkaline vegetables and stir-fry them in some olive oil for a while. Add in the tofu in the end and serve together.

Day 2 Plan

Breakfast

Apple parfait with coconut milk, raw cashews, green apple, uncooked oats, hemp seeds, and vanilla:

Put cashews, almond milk, and vanilla in a blender and mix until smooth. Layer the fixings in a little container. Add a stacking spoon of cashew cream, sliced apples, then add the oats with hemp seeds and eat!

Lunch

A savory avocado wrap made with butter lettuce, avocado, chopped basil, spinach, cilantro, onion, tomato, salt, and pepper:

Take the leaf and spread avocado on it. Then add basil and other ingredients over it. Fold the leaf equally, roll and enjoy!

Dinner

Tacos made with sweet potato and chickpea:

Opt for tacos made with alkaline grains if possible. Prepare some sweet potato and chickpeas by boiling them. Add these with other greens and some onion, lime and cilantro.

Day 3 Plan

Breakfast

Smoothie with almond milk, spinach, banana, chia seeds, strawberries, and almond butter:

Mix spinach and almond milk together first. At that point, include the remaining fixings except for chia, and mix. Include chia once all of it is smooth – at that point mix on an exceptionally low speed to blend. If there is no variable speed blender, blend chia in with the remainder of the fixings by hand. Let it sit for a couple of minutes so that the chia seeds can swell, and when they do, you can eat and enjoy.

Lunch

Zucchini pasta with kale, basil, olive oil, walnuts, lime, sea salt, pepper and cherry tomatoes:

The previous evening, soak the walnuts to improve assimilation into the mix. Put all the fixings in a blender or nourishment processor, and mix until you get a cream-like consistency. Add this over the zucchini noodles and it's done!

Dinner

Veggie wraps:

Prepare any vegetables you want and chop them up. Choose some leafy greens like lettuce or kale and wrap the vegetables in this. You can add some homemade hummus in this for added taste.

Day 4 Plan

Breakfast

Gluten-free oats with coconut milk, raw almond butter, green apple, and cinnamon:

Place the oats, coconut milk, and almond margarine into a bowl and blend well. Blend in the ground apple; use a covered bowl (or make your own using plastic wrap) and put in the fridge. Refrigerate for a few hours. If the oats get excessively thick, add some coconut milk to them. Top this with cinnamon powder.

Lunch

Salad with kale, broccoli, zucchini, kelp noodles, cherry tomatoes, hemp seeds, avocado, tahini, lemon, sea salt, cayenne pepper, and extra virgin olive oil:

Softly steam the kale and broccoli (preferably for 4 minutes), put aside. Blend zucchini noodles and kelp noodles and top with a generous serving of smoked avocado cumin dressing. Include cherry tomatoes and toss once more. Put the steamed kale and broccoli on a plate and drizzle them with lemon tahini dressing. Top kale and broccoli with the dressed noodles and tomatoes and sprinkle the entire dish with hemp seeds.

Dinner

Veggie burger with kale and sweet potato patty:

Boil some sweet potatoes and then mash them up once cool. Make them into patties and fry with olive oil. You can add some seasoning to the potato for taste. Once firm, wrap them in kale leaves and you have a burger ready.

Day 5 Plan

Breakfast

Smoothie made with almond milk, spinach, mixed berries, cinnamon, raw almond butter, banana, and coconut oil:

Mix spinach and almond milk first, at that point, include remaining fixings and mix well.

Lunch

Quinoa with black beans, green onions, lime, garlic, cumin, avocados, and some cilantro:

Cook the quinoa (or opt for brown rice). While cooking, warm the beans over a low flame. Mix in onions, lime juice, garlic, and cumin and let flavors consolidate for 10-15 minutes. At the point when quinoa is finished cooking, place it into individual serving bowls. Top with some beans, ripe avocado, and cilantro.

Dinner

Zucchini stir fry with beans:

You can opt for a standard or spiralized zucchini and any type of cooked beans you like. Just cook in ghee or coconut oil. Flavor your blend with mint, basil, cumin, garlic, thyme or onions. Include whatever else that will pan sear rapidly to make various varieties of this straightforward yet delectable concoction.

Day 6 Plan

Breakfast

Quinoa porridge with coconut milk, cinnamon, chia seeds, hemp seeds:

Mix all the fixings except hemp seeds and stew them for 10-15 minutes until the liquid is taken in. Top with hemp seeds.

The previous night, pour milk and chia seeds in a glass container. Include vanilla, cinnamon, and some nuts. Close with a top cover and shake the blend until it's thoroughly mixed. Refrigerate for a few hours. The following morning, shake or mix the blend and separate into two bowls. Top with a little crisp natural fruit, shredded coconut, and more chopped or crushed nuts.

Lunch

Thai salad made with quinoa, sesame seeds, garlic, lemon, and apple cider:

Vinegar, tamari, salt, arugula, tomato, onion, and sesame oil are the necessary ingredients.

In a blender, pour in filtered water and then the remainder of fixings. Mix. Steam some quinoa in a steamer or rice cooker, at that point put aside. Mix quinoa, arugula, cut tomatoes, diced red onion into a serving bowl, drizzle with the Thai dressing, and hand blend with a spoon before serving.

Dinner

Brussels sprouts with lemon and pistachios.

Warm 2 tbsp of unsalted, grass-fed butter in a skillet or a wok.

Include some pistachios and lemon zest. Sauté this for a minute or two. Add this around the shredded leaves of some Brussels sprouts (but don't use whole sprouts) and toss until it all looks green. Do this for around 5 minutes. Press out the juice from the lemon from which you got the zest and put in some salt and pepper or any different herbs you may prefer for taste. This delicious little treat is stacked with minerals and nutrients.

Day 7 Plan

Breakfast

Chia seed porridge with coconut milk, vanilla, cinnamon, coconut flakes, and chopped alkaline nuts:

The night before, pour milk and chia seeds together in a glass container. Add some vanilla, cinnamon powder and crushed nuts. Cover the container tightly and shake the blend until it's well-mixed. Refrigerate for the night. The following morning, shake or blend the mixtures and put into two serving bowls. Top with fresh organic fruit, shredded coconut or sliced nuts.

Lunch

Kelp noodles with scallion, sesame seeds, bell pepper, tahini, tamari, garlic, and coconut nectar:

In a salad bowl, blend all the dressing fixings and mix well with a spoon. For kelp noodles, soak them in some warm water for 10 minutes to flush off the fluid they are bundled with, allowing them to separate. Add the Asian sesame dressing to the noodles and scallions, and mix all ingredients together well. Sprinkle sesame seeds over this, and serve.

Dinner

Avocado salad with red onion and tomato:

The avocado should be diced into small pieces. Then, season it with some salt or pepper. In a different bowl, mix a diced tomato with ½ of a small red onion and another ½ of a jalapeño pepper. Also, add some of the finely cut-up cilantro or parsley. Include 2 tbsp of virgin olive oil, lemon juice and a pinch of cumin. Add and mix with the avocado chunks.

Snack Suggestions

Everyone wants a snack when they're hit with cravings or just a little hungry between meals. Stay away from the bag of chips and try some alkaline snacks instead.

- You can eat a ripe banana, as it is quite filling and rich in potassium.
- Try a few slices of any other fruit or a handful of alkaline-friendly nuts.
- If you're home and have time for an elaborate snack, you can make a small serving of avocado salad with hemp seeds and honey.
- Try a light smoothie with almond or coconut milk, kale, figs, and almond butter.

Do you still think that the alkaline diet could be boring or that you will have to suffer through flavorless meals? These are the kinds of meal plans that you need to prepare for yourself in the future. Just dedicate one day a week to meal planning and prepping. It will only take a little time to decide on the recipes you want for the week. Then you can cut and prep any ingredients you need (although be cautioned that avocados can oxidize if not used right away, leading them to turn dark and lose flavor). Use boxes that can be used for storing these ingredients in the fridge and use them as required. It's as simple as that. Most of these recipes don't even require cooking or baking so it will be even less time consuming than you might think.

It's okay if you can't avoid eating an unhealthy acidic meal once in a while. Don't pressure yourself to strive for total perfection. The alkaline diet does not require you to make big permanent promises to refrain from all the foods you like. Just try to keep the greasy burgers to a minimum and feed your body some healthy food to cut down on the acidic effects from those acidifying foods. It's as simple as finding the right balance.

A nutritionist can help you create your alkaline diet plan if you have any particular health issues that need to be taken into consideration. You may even take guidance from an expert to create a meal plan that will help you treat certain conditions or improve your health; however, it is not necessary. The plan given here is simple enough (and tasty, too!), and you can easily make your own plans after you get through the first week. You can even switch out meals from this plan with any other recipe you want to try from the book. There are no restrictions because these are all alkaline-friendly foods that will improve your health.

Chapter Nine: Cleansing The Body

You can jumpstart the healing effect of the alkaline diet by carrying out a few short cleansing techniques with the body parts that are most affected by acidic diets.

Colon Cleansing

One important organ in the digestive framework is the colon, also known as the large intestine. Colon health is a unique piece of digestional well-being. A few people insist the colon ought to be purged for ideal health within the digestive system. Be that as it may, investigations demonstrating the effectiveness of such purifications and cleanses are sparse and low in quality. In any case, certain parts of colon purging might be advantageous. It might help alleviate certain issues, for example, blockages in the intestines or sporadic bowel movements, and there is some proof that they can likewise diminish the risk of developing colon cancer. Other colon-cleanse-related claims, however, are flawed-- for example, removal of poisons and parasites. There are a couple of approaches to colon cleansing. You can buy a colon-cleansing product at a drug store or online, or you can even get a colonic water enema or similar colon irrigation system.

Otherwise, you can do basic things to support or "wash down" the digestive tract and practice good colon health at home.

The regular colon rinses we will discuss here can be efficiently done for a low cost, and they're very safe when done the right way.

Water Flush

Drinking a lot of water and remaining

hydrated is a wonderful method for ensuring colon health and digestive health overall. Individuals who suggest a water flush for colon purification suggest drinking six to eight glasses of tepid water every day. This helps with overall hydration, too, which benefits health in many ways as previously discussed.

Salt Water Flush

You can also attempt a salt water flush. This is particularly useful for individuals encountering bowel obstruction and inconsistency with bowel movements. A recent report showed that salt water could clear the colon when matched with certain yoga practices. Before eating in the first part of the day, blend two teaspoons salt with tepid water. Ocean salt or Himalayan salt is the best for this. Drink water rapidly on an empty stomach, and in no time flat, you'll most likely feel the urge to go to the restroom. Do this toward the beginning of the day, and make a point to remain at home close to the restroom for some time after the cleansing. You may need to go to the restroom on multiple occasions. Additionally, have a go at eating a lot of food that is high in water content. This includes delicious foods like watermelons, tomatoes, lettuce, cucumber, and celery. There are a lot of nourishing foods that can assist in cleansing the colon through an eating regimen.

High Fiber Diet

Fiber is a fundamental macronutrient regularly neglected in the modern-day eating regimen. It's found in whole foods like natural products, vegetables, grains, nuts, seeds, and the sky's the limit from there. Plants contain a lot of cellulose with fiber that assists in the mass accumulation of waste matter in the colon. They likewise keep bowel obstruction and overactive guts in check, while boosting accommodating microbes as a prebiotic. Make a point to eat a lot of high-fiber foods, which help maintain a solid colon. They can also be incredible for managing bacteria in the gut.

Drink More Juices

Juices are well-known colon cleansers. Incorporate leafy vegetable juice fasts and cleanses, similar to a purge. There isn't sufficient research on these for the colon, though, to advise these on a regular basis. Some research shows that there are potential hazards to doing too many juice cleanses. All things being equal, moderate consumption of juices and squeezes can be beneficial for you. Juice mixes contain some fiber and supplements that boost metabolic processing. They also have water in them that can help hydrate and keep up regularity of the digestive system. Furthermore, a study from 2015 found that vitamin C might be helpful in the purification of the colon. This nutrient is found in a variety of leafy foods that are often added to juice mixes.

Side effects of a colon cleanse might include nausea, vomiting, dizziness, dehydration and cramping and electrolyte imbalance. Stop the cleanse if you experience any of these symptoms. Consult your physician and ensure that it is safe if you still want to continue. There is rarely any risk involved in a colon cleanse, but it is better to be safe than sorry; however, engaging in frequent colon cleansing can be harmful and cause bowel injury or chronic constipation.

Kidney Cleanse

The kidneys are two little organs located on

either side of the spine, underneath the ribs. They play a significant part in disposing of bodily wastes, adjusting electrolytes, and producing hormones. As long as there is no additional illness, a balanced eating routine and sufficient water consumption are generally enough to keep your kidneys healthy. Be that as it may, certain supplements, herbs, and dietary enhancements can help in boosting kidney function.

Hydration

The human body is made up of nearly 60 percent water. Every organ, from the cerebrum to the liver, needs water to be able to work. As the filtration organ of the body, the kidneys need water in order for the body to emit urine. Urine is a critical waste product that enables the body to dispose of undesirable or superfluous substances. At the point when water hydration is low, urine volume is also low. A low urine yield may be accompanied by kidney dysfunction, for example, the creation of kidney stones. It's vital to drink enough water so that the kidneys can appropriately flush out any abundance of waste materials. This is particularly significant for a kidney cleanse.

Foods Supporting Kidney Health

Here is a list of some foods that support kidney health:

- Grapes, peanuts, and a few berries contain an important plant compound called resveratrol. In one animal study[17], specialists found that treatment with resveratrol could bring down kidney irritation in rodents with polycystic kidney ailment.

---

[17] Kitada, M., & Koya, D. (2013). Renal protective effects of resveratrol. *Oxidative medicine and cellular longevity, 2013*, 568093. doi:10.1155/2013/568093

- Cranberries have regularly been applauded for their benefits related to bladder function. A clinical study[18] in the *Nutrition Journal* showed that females who ate dried cranberries every day for about fourteen days encountered a diminishing effect in the frequency of urinary tract problems.

- Brown seaweed is considered good for the pancreas, kidneys, and liver. In a 2014 animal preliminary study, rodents consumed edible seaweed for a time of 22 days and demonstrated a decrease in both kidney and liver harm from diabetes.

---

[18] Burleigh, A. E., Benck, S. M., McAchran, S. E., Reed, J. D., Krueger, C. G., & Hopkins, W. J. (2013). Consumption of sweetened, dried cranberries may reduce urinary tract infection incidence in susceptible women--a modified observational study. *Nutrition journal, 12*(1), 139. doi:10.1186/1475-2891-12-139

Chapter Ten: FAQ About The Alkaline Diet

By now you should know enough about the alkaline diet to help you get started. This section will help you clear any lingering doubts and answer any remaining questions. The following are all the frequently asked questions on these topics and some questions that we anticipate readers may have. I hope you find the answers clear and informative.

What Are Alkaline Forming Foods?

Alkaline forming foods are those that form alkaline products after they have been broken down inside the body. Certain foods are acid forming because, after digestion, the end product ends up as an acidic substance within the body.

How Do Alkaline Foods Help?

Alkaline foods will help to restore a healthy pH level in the body to ensure well-being. They will help to neutralize excess acids that are obtained from other foods and reduce the risk of inflammation or other diseases. Cutting back on acid forming foods and replacing them with alkaline forming foods can result in positive benefits for your body and health.

Is The Alkaline Diet Gluten Free ?

The diet is not specifically gluten free. Certain foods that contain gluten are cut out of the diet so you can still follow it as a gluten-free diet by making your own adjustments.

Are The Ingredients For This Diet Expensive?

The alkaline diet is not made up of fancy expensive ingredients that you will need to spend exorbitant amounts of money on. You need to get rid of the unhealthy food from your pantry and stock it with healthy produce. Stock up on fresh fruits and vegetables, herbs, spices, and other wholesome foods, and you're good to go.

Is The Alkaline Diet A Completely Vegetarian Diet?

No, the diet does not require you to give up meat if you don't want to. It just suggests that you reduce the amount of meat you consume and replace it with more fruits and vegetables. Excessive meat consumption induces acid formation in the body. The protein in the diet will be abundantly provided by lentils, nuts, seeds, and other sources. Try to keep 80% of your diet alkaline while the rest (20%) can be acidic and include meat. Although most of the recipes in the alkaline diet are free of meat, you can find a balanced way to include them if you so desire.

Will The Diet Help With Acid Reflux?

Yes. Alkaline foods will help to reduce the symptoms of and even aid in preventing acid reflux over time. One of the easiest ways to prevent acid reflux is drinking alkaline water. It will reduce indigestion and reduce stomach acid too. Also, try to avoid any foods that cause acid reflux in your body in the first place.

Will It Help With Weight Loss?

The alkaline diet is not designed for helping you with quick weight loss; however, it is a healthy diet filled with low-calorie and high-fiber foods. This factor will help with losing weight if you combine it with an active lifestyle. Don't expect any quick results but the alkaline diet will surely help you eat healthily and reduce excess weight.

How Long Does It Take For The Body Acids To Be Neutralized?

There is no fixed answer for this. Most of us have been following the acid-forming modern diet for a long time, and the impact of it is therefore long-standing. Each person's body can take a different amount of time to become alkaline again. No complete change will happen in a short time and last forever. It would be best if you aimed to follow the diet in a way that you can keep a balanced pH level over time; however, the subtle effects of the diet can be felt within a couple of days of beginning the diet. You will see that you sleep better and your energy levels will become more stable.

Do I Have To Eat Only Raw Food?

No, you don't. Cooking can reduce the nutrient value of foods, but you can continue to cook. Try to steam certain foods and eat foods like fruits raw as much as possible. This will allow you to get the most of the essential vitamins and minerals in your food.

Will It Help Gout?

When there is uric acid build up in the body, it leads to gout. Lowering uric acid levels is possible on an alkaline diet. This should help in the prevention of gout attacks. Food triggers that stimulate gout attacks can be easily avoided on an alkaline diet.

Will It Help In Diabetes?

Yes, alkaline forming foods tend to help to regulate blood pressure. Most alkaline foods don't cause blood sugar spikes, unlike foods in the modern diet. A specialized diet for diabetics is usually full of alkaline forming foods anyway. You can try this diet to help you lower your risk for diabetes to a large extent. You can always ask your doctor first.

Is The Diet Safe For The Whole Family To Follow?

Yes! The alkaline diet can be followed and should be followed by everyone from adults to children in your household. It is a balanced diet that promotes good health by increasing consumption of nutritional food. You don't have to cook separately for yourself while cooking other meals for your family. Everyone can enjoy the benefits of this diet.

Is The Alkaline Diet Very Time-Consuming?

One of the worst habits of the modern generation is that they do not set aside time for important meals. It is worth the time and effort to invest in preparing good healthy food to ensure long-term good health. Meal prepping is one of the easiest tricks to save time if you have a busy lifestyle. Just prep ingredients once a week and you only have to put them together when you eat. Thank goodness for refrigerators!

Will The Alkaline Diet Help With Acne?

An acidic diet can have many side effects and acne is one of them. This is due to the fact that the greasy fast food in the modern diet promotes acne; however, switching to an alkaline diet will counteract this and help to reduce breakouts. The antioxidants and vitamins from this diet will help you achieve glowing skin that is healthy over time.

Most of your questions should have been answered in this section. If you have any more, you can probably find the answers in the rest of the book or look it up online. But I assure you, the alkaline diet is a sure bet for good health over the long term.

Chapter Eleven: Alkaline Smoothie Recipes

Green Alkaline Smoothie[19]

Serves: 2

Ingredients:

- 2 avocados, peeled, pitted, chopped
- Juice of 2 lemons
- 10-12 leaves kale, discard hard stems and ribs
- ½ small cucumber, sliced
- 2 cups raw almond milk
- ¼ teaspoons ground cinnamon
- A handful mint leaves

Method:

---

[19] Alkaline Smoothie Recipes - Holistic Wellness Project. (2019). Retrieved from https://www.holisticwellnessproject.com/blog/alkaline-diet/amazing-alkaline-smoothies/

1. Blend together all the ingredients in a blender until smooth.

2. Pour into glasses and serve.

Grapefruit Smoothie20

Serves: 2

Ingredients:

- 2 cups spinach
- 2 cups coconut milk
- Juice of 2 grapefruits
- Stevia to taste
- Ice cubes, as required

Method:

1. Blend together all the ingredients in a blender until smooth.

2. Pour into glasses and serve.

---

[20] Alkaline Smoothie Recipes - Holistic Wellness Project. (2019). Retrieved from https://www.holisticwellnessproject.com/blog/alkaline-diet/amazing-alkaline-smoothies/

Anti-Inflammation Smoothie21

Serves: 4

Ingredients:

- 2 inches fresh ginger, peeled, grated
- 1 cup baby spinach
- 1 large avocado, peeled pitted, chopped
- 1 cup flat-leaf parsley or cilantro
- ¼ teaspoon cayenne pepper
- 2 inches fresh turmeric, peeled, grated
- Handful watercress or rocket lettuce or arugula
- 1 bell pepper, deseeded, chopped
- 2 cups coconut water or filtered water
- A pinch salt

---

[21] Alkaline Recipe #166: The Anti-Inflammatory Smoothie - Live Energized. (2019). Retrieved from https://liveenergized.com/alkaline-recipes/alkaline-recipe-166-anti-inflammatory-smoothie/

Method:

1. Blend together all the ingredients in a blender until smooth.
2. Pour into glasses and serve.

Veggie Blast Smoothie22

Serves: 2-3

Ingredients:

- 2 cucumbers, peeled, sliced
- 2 cloves garlic, peeled
- 1 cup rosemary infused water, cooled
- 2 tablespoons virgin olive oil
- Juice of 2 lemons
- 8 tomatoes, peeled, chopped
- 1 onion, chopped
- Pepper to taste

---

22 Alkaline Smoothie Recipes - Holistic Wellness Project. (2019). Retrieved from https://www.holisticwellnessproject.com/blog/alkaline-diet/amazing-alkaline-smoothies/

- Himalayan pink salt to taste
- 2 cups spinach or kale juice
- Pumpkin seeds, to garnish

Method:

1. Blend together cucumber, garlic, tomato, onion and olive oil in a blender until smooth.

2. Pour into a jug. Add rest of the ingredients and stir.

3. Pour into glasses and serve garnished with pumpkin seeds.

Pomegranate Smoothie23

Serves: 2-3

Ingredients:

---

[23] Alkaline Smoothie Recipes - Holistic Wellness Project. (2019). Retrieved from https://www.holisticwellnessproject.com/blog/alkaline-diet/amazing-alkaline-smoothies/

- 4 grapefruits, peeled, deseeded
- 6 large collard leaves, discard stems
- 1 cup pomegranate arils
- 2 cups coconut water

Method:

1. Blend together all the ingredients in a blender until smooth.
2. Pour into glasses and serve.

Nut And Seed Smoothie[24]

Serves: 4

Ingredients:

- 1 avocado, peeled, pitted, chopped
- 4 handfuls watercress, kale or greens of your choice
- 4 handful baby spinach
- 1 cup almonds soaked in water for 7-8 hours.
- 2 cups almond milk, unsweetened
- 2 tablespoons almond butter
- 2 tablespoons coconut oil
- 2 cups water
- 2 tablespoons chia seeds, to serve

Method:

1. Blend together all the ingredients in

---

[24] The Smoothie That Keeps You Going Until Lunch - Live Energized. (2019). Retrieved from https://liveenergized.com/alkaline-diet-resources/the-smoothie-that-keeps-you-going-until-lunch/

a blender until smooth.

2. Pour into glasses. Add ½ tablespoon chia seeds into each glass and stir.

3. Let it sit for a few minutes to swell up before serving.

Avocado Power Smoothie25

Serves: 4

Ingredients:

- 2 cucumbers, chopped
- 2 avocados, peeled, pitted, chopped
- 4 tomatoes, chopped
- 2 handfuls spinach leaves
- 1 red bell pepper, chopped
- Juice of a lime
- 2 tablespoons vegetable stock

Optional: Use any

---

25 Alkaline Recipe #23 Alkaline Avocado Power Shake - Live Energized. (2019). Retrieved from https://liveenergized.com/alkaline-recipes/alkaline-recipe-23-alkaline-avocado-power-shake/

- 2 scoops super soy sprouts (optional)
- 1 scoop Mega greens powder
- Lettuce leaves or kale
- Ground ginger
- Ground cumin
- Ground cumin
- Fresh herbs of your choice

Method:

1. Add all the ingredients to the blender and blend until smooth.

2. Pour in tall glasses and serve with crushed ice.

Sweet And Chunky Shake26

Serves: 4

Ingredients:

- 2 cucumbers, chopped
- 2 avocados, peeled, pitted, chopped
- 8 tomatoes, chopped
- 4 stalks celery, chopped
- 4 small heads broccoli with stalks, chopped
- 2 red bell peppers, deseeded, chopped
- Juice of a lime
- 5-6 tablespoons vegetable stock mixed with 5-6 tablespoons warm water
- A handful fresh basil

Method:

---

[26] Alkaline Recipe #27 Sweet Chunky Alkaline Shake! - Live Energized. (2019). Retrieved from https://liveenergized.com/alkaline-recipes/alkaline-recipe-26-sweet-chunky-alkaline-shake/

1. Add stock and avocado into a blender and blend until smooth.

2. Add rest of the ingredients and pulse until slightly chunky in texture.

3. Pour into glasses and serve.

Green Smoothie27

Serves: 2-3

Ingredients:

- 2 medium cucumbers, chopped
- ¼ cup fresh mint leaves
- 2 inches fresh ginger, peeled, sliced
- 2 cups coconut water
- 2-3 teaspoons udo's oil
- 4-5 drops stevia or 2 teaspoons agave nectar
- 6 kale leaves, remove the hard

27 Alkaline Smoothie Recipes - Holistic Wellness Project. (2019). Retrieved from https://www.holisticwellnessproject.com/blog/alkaline-diet/amazing-alkaline-smoothies/

stems and ribs, torn

- 2 avocados, peeled, pitted, chopped
- 6 stalks fresh parsley, chopped
- 2-3 tablespoons hemp seeds
- Juice of a lime

Method:

1. Add all the ingredients to the blender and blend until smooth.

2. Pour in tall glasses and serve with crushed ice.

Banana Chocolate Smoothie28

Serves: 2

Ingredients:

- 2 large bananas, sliced, frozen
- 4 teaspoons cacao powder

---

[28] Oaxaca Chocolate Banana Smoothie Recipe - Cookie and Kate. (2019). Retrieved from https://cookieandkate.com/oaxaca-chocolate-banana-smoothie/

- A pinch cayenne pepper (optional)
- 1 ½ cups cashew milk or any other plant based milk of your choice
- 2 tablespoons dark chocolate chips
- ½ teaspoon ground cinnamon
- 1 teaspoon maple syrup or honey (optional)
- 2 tablespoons sliced, toasted almonds, to garnish (optional)

Method:

1. Add all the ingredients to the blender and blend until smooth.

2. Pour in tall glasses. Sprinkle almonds on top and serve with crushed ice.

Chapter Twelve: Alkaline Breakfast Recipes

Avocado Breakfast Salad29

Serves: 3-4

Ingredients:

- 4 tortillas, chopped into bite size pieces
- 2 avocados, peeled, pitted, chopped
- ½ cup chopped almonds
- 2 teaspoons chili sauce
- 1 red onion, sliced
- 1 package firm tofu, chopped into cubes
- 2 pink grapefruits, peeled, separated into segments, chopped

---

[29] 10 Healthy Alkaline Breakfast Recipes You Must Try. (2019). Retrieved from https://medium.com/@dietauthority/10-healthy-alkaline-breakfast-recipes-you-must-try-4e91fcf4731b

- 8 handfuls baby spinach
- 4 tomatoes, chopped
- Juice of a lemon

Method:

1. Bake in a preheated oven at 350º F until crisp.

2. Add tofu, tomatoes, chili sauce and onions into a bowl and toss well. Chill for a couple of hours.

3. Add lemon juice, grapefruits, avocado and almonds and toss well.

4. Divide into plates. Scatter crisp tortilla pieces on top and serve.

Kale Chickpea Mash[30]

Serves: 4-5

Ingredients:

- 2 cans (14.1 ounces each) chickpeas, rinsed, drained
- 6 tablespoons minced garlic
- 2 bunches kale, discard hard ribs and stems, chopped
- 2 shallots, chopped
- 4 tablespoons coconut oil
- Salt to taste

Method:

1. Place a skillet over medium heat. Add oil. When oil melts, add onion and garlic. Sauté until onions are golden brown.

---

[30] 10 Healthy Alkaline Breakfast Recipes You Must Try. (2019). Retrieved from https://medium.com/@dietauthority/10-healthy-alkaline-breakfast-recipes-you-must-try-4e91fcf4731b

2. Add kale and sauté until the kale wilts. Add chickpeas and cook for a while.

3. Mash with a fork to the consistency you desire and serve.

Quinoa and Apple Breakfast31

Serves: 2

Ingredients:

- 1 cup quinoa
- Juice of a lemon
- 2 apples, peeled, grated
- 1 teaspoon ground cinnamon
- 2 cups water
- Raisins to serve (optional)

Method:

---

[31] 10 Healthy Alkaline Breakfast Recipes You Must Try. (2019). Retrieved from https://medium.com/@dietauthority/10-healthy-alkaline-breakfast-recipes-you-must-try-4e91fcf4731b

1. Add water and quinoa into a saucepan. Place saucepan over medium heat.

2. When the mixture begins to boil, lower the heat and simmer until nearly dry.

3. Add apples and cook for about a minutes.

4. Serve in bowls, garnished with cinnamon.

5. Serve with raisins (if using) or any other alkaline-friendly toppings of your choice.

Scrambled Tofu32

Serves: 3

Ingredients:

---

32 10 Healthy Alkaline Breakfast Recipes You Must Try. (2019). Retrieved from https://medium.com/@dietauthority/10-healthy-alkaline-breakfast-recipes-you-must-try-4e91fcf4731b

- 2 – 2 ½ cups crumbled firm tofu
- 3 tomatoes, chopped
- 1 onion, chopped
- 1 tablespoon olive or coconut oil
- 2 cups baby spinach
- 2 cloves garlic, sliced
- Paprika to taste
- ¼ teaspoon turmeric
- 1 teaspoon ground cumin
- Freshly ground pepper to taste
- Salt to taste

Method:

1. Place a skillet over medium heat. Add oil and let it heat. Add onions and sauté until the onions are translucent. Add turmeric and cumin and sauté for 5-10 seconds.

2. Add tomatoes, salt, pepper, paprika and tofu. Sprinkle some water as well.

Sauté for 3-4 minutes.

3. Garnish with some fresh herbs of your choice if desired and serve.

Quinoa Porridge33

Serves: 2

Ingredients:

- 1 cup quinoa
- 2 tablespoons coconut oil
- ½ teaspoon ground cinnamon
- 2 tablespoons chia seeds
- ½ cup plant based milk
- ½ teaspoon stevia extract
- 2 ½ cups + 1/3 cup water
- Walnuts or hemp seeds to top

Method:

1. Place chia seeds in a bowl. Pour

---

33 Marks, E. (2019). 12 Easy and Delicious Alkaline Breakfast Recipes For Energy. Retrieved from https://great4you.co/alkaline-breakfast-recipes/

about 1/3 cup water and let it soak for at least 15 minutes.

2. Add quinoa and 2 ½ cups water into a saucepan. Place the saucepan over medium heat. Bring to a boil.

3. Lower the heat and simmer until nearly dry.

4. Add rest of the ingredients and stir.

5. Ladle into bowls. Serve garnished with hemp seeds or walnuts.

Warm Blueberry Porridge34

Serves: 2

Ingredients:

- ½ cup buckwheat groats, soaked in water overnight, drained, rinsed well
- 20 almonds, chopped
- ½ teaspoon ground cinnamon

---

34 Marks, E. (2019). 12 Easy and Delicious Alkaline Breakfast Recipes For Energy. Retrieved from https://great4you.co/alkaline-breakfast-recipes/

- Stevia drops to taste
- 2 tablespoons chia seeds
- 1 cup almond milk, unsweetened
- ½ teaspoon vanilla extract
- Blueberries to serve

Method:

1. Add chia seeds and almonds into a bowl. Pour about a cup of water. Cover and set aside overnight.

2. Add almond milk and buckwheat groats into a nonstick skillet. Place skillet over medium heat. Cook until they crack and the mixture is creamy.

3. Add rest of the ingredients and stir.

4. Heat thoroughly.

5. Serve in bowls. Sprinkle blueberries on top and serve.

Chocolate Chia Pudding35

Serves: 2

Ingredients:

- ½ cup chia seeds
- 3 tablespoons cacao powder
- ¼ teaspoon ground cinnamon
- 2 ½ cups plant based milk
- 2 teaspoons vanilla extract
- ¼ teaspoon sea salt
- ½ teaspoon stevia extract

Method:

1. Add chia seeds, cacao powder, cinnamon, milk, vanilla, salt and stevia into a bowl. Stir until well combined.
2. Cover and chill for 5-6 hours.
3. Stir and serve in bowls.

Sprouted Buckwheat Crepes[36]

[35] Marks, E. (2019). 12 Easy and Delicious Alkaline Breakfast Recipes For Energy. Retrieved from https://great4you.co/alkaline-breakfast-recipes/
[36] Marks, E. (2019). 12 Easy and Delicious Alkaline Breakfast Recipes For

Serves: 8

Ingredients:

- 2 cups buckwheat groats, rinsed a few times, soaked in 4 cups water overnight
- 2 tablespoons chia seeds
- 1 ½ cups water
- 2 tablespoons pure vanilla extract
- Coconut oil, to fry
- Sprouted nut butter, or hemp seeds or any other toppings of your choice

Method:

1. Drain and rinse the buckwheat well (after soaking overnight).

2. Add all the ingredients into a blender and blend until smooth.

3. Place a nonstick pan over medium-high heat. Add about 1 teaspoon oil and

Energy. Retrieved from https://great4you.co/alkaline-breakfast-recipes/

swirl the pan so that the oil spreads.

4. Pour about ¼ cup of the blended mixture on the heated pan. Swirl the pan so that the batter spreads slightly.

5. When the underside is cooked, flip sides and cook the other side.

6. Slide the crepe onto a plate.

7. Repeat steps 3-6 and make the remaining crepes. Serve with the suggested toppings.

Healthier Baked Beans37

Serves: 3

Ingredients:

- 2 cups organic butter beans, rinsed a few times, drained
- ½ white onion, diced
- 2 teaspoons dry mustard powder
- 2 teaspoons coconut oil
- Sea salt to taste
- 2 drops liquid stevia
- Few avocado slices, to serve
- 4 tablespoons tomato paste
- 2 cloves garlic, sliced
- 1 teaspoon smoked paprika
- 1 cup halved cherry tomatoes
- Cracked pepper to taste
- 2 cups fresh baby spinach

---

[37] Marks, E. (2019). 12 Easy and Delicious Alkaline Breakfast Recipes For Energy. Retrieved from https://great4you.co/alkaline-breakfast-recipes/

Method:

1. Place a pan over medium-low heat. Add oil. When the oil melts, add onion and garlic and sauté until translucent.

2. Stir in butter beans, tomato paste and tomatoes; simmer for 3-4 minutes.

3. Add paprika, salt, pepper, mustard and stevia and mix well.

4. Divide into plates. Top with spinach and avocado slices and serve.

Sprouted Toast w/ Cherry Tomatoes, Avocado, and Hemp Oil[38]

Serves: 2

Ingredients:

- 2 slices sprouted Ezekiel bread, toasted
- A handful cherry tomatoes, halved
- Avocado slices, as required
- Hemp oil, to drizzle
- Pepper to taste
- Salt to taste

Method:

1. Place the toasted bread slices on a serving platter. Spread the avocado slices over it.

---

[38]Marks, E. (2019). 12 Easy and Delicious Alkaline Breakfast Recipes For Energy. Retrieved from https://great4you.co/alkaline-breakfast-recipes/

2. Scatter cherry tomatoes. Season with salt and pepper. Drizzle oil and serve.

Chapter Thirteen: Alkaline Snacks

Energy Crackers with Hummus39

Serves: 20-25

Ingredients:

- 1 cup chia seeds
- 1 cup pumpkin seeds
- 2 cloves garlic, peeled, crushed
- Salt to taste
- Pepper to taste
- 1 cup sesame seeds
- 1 cup sunflower seeds
- 1 teaspoon cayenne pepper
- 2 ½ cups water

---

[39] 11 High Protein, Portable, Alkaline Snacks - Live Energized. (2019). Retrieved from https://liveenergized.com/alkaline-diet-tips/11-high-protein-portable-alkaline-snacks/

Method:

1. Add all the ingredients into a large bowl and stir. Let it sit for 10 minutes.

2. Line a large baking sheet with parchment paper.

3. Spread the mixture on the baking sheet. Cut into 20-25 equal squares.

4. Bake in a preheated oven at 300°F for 30 minutes. Flip sides and bake for another 20-25 minutes or until golden brown.

Toasted Quinoa Bites[40]

Serves: Makes 20-25 bites

Ingredients:

- 1 cup quinoa
- ½ cup pumpkin seeds

---

[40] 11 High Protein, Portable, Alkaline Snacks - Live Energized. (2019). Retrieved from https://liveenergized.com/alkaline-diet-tips/11-high-protein-portable-alkaline-snacks/

- 1 teaspoon ground cinnamon
- ½ cup shredded coconut
- 2 tablespoons ground flax seeds
- 1 teaspoon ground cinnamon
- Rice malt syrup, as required

Method:

1. Add all the ingredients except rice malt syrup into a baking dish. Stir until well combined.

2. Pour some rice malt syrup into the baking dish and stir until well combined. The mixture should be spreadable but not runny. Cut into 20-25 pieces.

3. Bake in a preheated oven at 425 °F for 10-12 minutes or until crisp. Be careful as it can get burnt.

Superfood Protein Balls[41]

[41] 11 High Protein, Portable, Alkaline Snacks - Live Energized. (2019). Retrieved from https://liveenergized.com/alkaline-diet-tips/11-high-protein-portable-alkaline-snacks/

Serves: Makes 25-30 balls

Ingredients:

- 1 cup almonds
- 2/3 cup walnuts
- 2/3 cup chia seeds
- ½ cup coconut palm sugar
- 2/3 cup pepitas (pumpkin seeds)
- ½ cup black sesame seeds
- 1 cup tahini
- ½ cup almond butter

Method:

1. Add all the ingredients into the food processor bowl.

2. Process until coarsely ground and well combined.

3. Divide the mixture into 25-30 equal portions and shape into balls.

4. Store in an airtight container in the

refrigerator until use.

Best Peanut Butter Protein Ball42

Serves: Makes 15-20 balls

Ingredients:

- 2 cups rolled oats
- 2 tablespoons flax seeds or chia seeds
- 1 teaspoon ground cinnamon
- 1 ½ teaspoons stevia extract
- 1 cup 100% pure peanut butter
- 2 teaspoons vanilla extract
- 2/3 cup dark chocolate chunks
- 6 tablespoons water

Method:

1. Add oats, cinnamon, flaxseeds and stevia into a bowl and stir.

---

42 Marks, E. (2019). 18 Healthy "No Bake" Protein Ball Recipes (Updated). Retrieved from https://great4you.co/protein-ball-recipes/

2. Stir in the vanilla and peanut butter.

3. Add chocolate chips and stir until well incorporated. Add water, a tablespoon at a time and mix well each time. Add enough such that you are able to form into balls.

4. Divide the mixture into 15-20 equal portions and shape into balls.

5. Chill and serve.

Avocado French Fries[43]

Serves: 4-6

Ingredients:

- 3-4 Hass avocados, peeled, pitted, cut into fries

For parmesan:

- 1-2 teaspoons sea salt to taste
- 5-6 tablespoons sesame seeds

Method:

1. To make "parmesan": Add sesame seeds and salt in a spice grinder or coffee grinder and grind into a powder. Transfer into a large bowl.

2. Add avocado pieces and toss until well coated.

---

[43] Alkaline Diet Recipe: Avocado French Fries. (2019). Retrieved from https://www.getoffyouracid.com/blogs/snacks/alkaline-diet-recipe-avocado-french-fries

3. Place on a lined baking sheet.

4. Bake in a preheated oven at 300°F for about 15-20 minutes or until crisp. Stir once halfway through baking.

Zucchini "Tater" Tots44

Serves: 5-6

Ingredients:

- 3-4 small potatoes, cooked, grated
- Salt to taste
- Pepper to taste
- Sweet paprika to taste
- 1 medium zucchini, grated, squeezed of excess moisture
- Olive oil, to brush

Method:

1. Add all the ingredients into a bowl and mix well.

2. Make 20-25 equal portions and shape into tater tots (small cylindrical shapes).

3. Place on a lined baking sheet, in a

---

44 Zucchini Tater Tots [Vegan]. (2019). Retrieved from
https://www.onegreenplanet.org/vegan-recipe/zucchini-tater-tots/

single layer. Brush all over the tater tots with oil.

4. Bake in a preheated oven at 425°F for 30-40 minutes or until crisp.

5. Serve hot with your favorite alkaline-friendly dip.

Celery With Nut Butter45

Serves: 4-6

Ingredients:

- 4-6 sticks celery
- Seeds of your choice like chia seeds, sesame seeds, etc. toasted (optional)
- Almond butter, as required

Method:

1. Fill the celery sticks with almond

---

[45] Alkaline Snacks: The Ultimate List of Alkaline Snacks & Recipes. (2019). Retrieved from https://liveenergized.com/alkaline-diet-resources/alkaline-snacks/

butter.

2. Sprinkle seeds on it and serve.

Veggie Sticks With Quick & Easy Tahini46

Serves: 4-6

Ingredients:

- 4 tablespoons raw organic tahini
- 2 teaspoons fresh lemon juice
- 2 squirts liquid aminos
- Chili powder to taste
- Vegetable sticks (like carrot, cucumber, celery, cut into sticks), as required

Method:

---

[46] Snack Attack - Great Ideas for a Healthy, Alkaline & Beautiful Body - Living Pretty, Naturally. (2019). Retrieved from http://livingprettynaturally.com/why-alkaline-body-is-important-healthy-snacks-for-beauty/

1. Add tahini, lemon juice, aminos and chili powder into a bowl and mix well.

2. Serve with vegetable sticks.

Kale Chips47

Serves: 5-6

Ingredients:

- 2-3 large bunch curly kale leaves, discard hard stems and ribs, tear the leaves into large pieces
- Sea salt to taste
- 1-2 tablespoons coconut oil

Method:

1. Add kale leaves into large bowl. Sprinkle salt and drizzle oil. Toss well so as to coat the leaves.

---

47 Snack Attack - Great Ideas for a Healthy, Alkaline & Beautiful Body - Living Pretty, Naturally. (2019). Retrieved from http://livingprettynaturally.com/why-alkaline-body-is-important-healthy-snacks-for-beauty/

2. Spread the leaves on 1-2 baking sheets.

3. Bake in a preheated oven at 350 °F for about 10 minutes or until crisp.

4. Store in an airtight container.

Chopped Berries With Mint And Coconut Butter48

Serves: 2-3

Ingredients:

- 2 cups mixed berries of your choice
- 2 tablespoons chopped mint leaves
- 4 tablespoons coconut butter, melted

Method:

1. Add berries and mint into a bowl

---

48 Chopped Berries with Mint and Coconut Butter. (2019). Retrieved from https://www.getoffyouracid.com/blogs/desserts/chopped-berries-with-mint-and-coconut-butter

and toss well.

2. Divide into 2-3 bowls. Drizzle melted coconut butter on top and serve.

Alkaline Brazil Nut Cheese49

Makes: About 2 cups

Ingredients:

- ½ pound Brazil nuts, soaked in water overnight
- 1 teaspoon sea salt
- ¼ teaspoon cayenne pepper
- ¾ cup water
- 1 teaspoon lime juice
- ½ teaspoon onion powder
- ¾ cup hemp milk
- 1 teaspoon grape seed oil

Method:

---

49 Alkaline Electric Brazil Nut Cheese - Ty's Conscious Kitchen. (2019). Retrieved from https://www.tysconsciouskitchen.com/dr-sebi-alkaline-electric-brazil-nut-cheese/

1. Add all the ingredients into a blender except water. Blend for a minute. Add ¼ cup water at a time and blend well each time until the consistency you desire is achieved.

2. Enjoy as it is or serve with sandwiches, zucchini pasta, burgers etc.

Chapter Fourteen: Alkaline Salads And Soups

Kale Quinoa Salad With Lemon Vinaigrette[50]

Serves: 8

Ingredients:

<u>For salad:</u>

- 8 cups chopped kale, discard hard ribs and stems
- 1 cup cooked quinoa
- 1 cup chopped almonds
- 1 cup pomegranate arils
- 2 avocados, peeled, pitted, cubed

<u>For lemon vinaigrette dressing:</u>

---

[50] Kale Quinoa Salad with Lemon Vinaigrette. (2019). Retrieved from https://www.getoffyouracid.com/blogs/salads/kale-quinoa-salad-with-lemon-vinaigrette

- ½ cup apple cider vinegar
- Zest of 2 lemons, grated
- ½ cup extra-virgin olive oil
- Salt to taste (sea salt or Himalayan pink salt)
- Freshly ground pepper to taste
- 6 tablespoons fresh lemon juice

Method:

1. To make lemon vinaigrette dressing: Add all the ingredients of dressing into a small jar. Fasten with lid. Shake vigorously. Set aside for a while for the flavors to blend in.
2. Add all the ingredients for salad in a bowl and toss well. Pour dressing on top.
3. Toss well and serve.

Quinoa Salad With Avocados[51]

Serves: 6-8

Ingredients:

- 2 cucumbers, peeled, chopped
- 6 Roma tomatoes, deseeded, finely chopped
- 3 cups quinoa
- ½ cup extra-virgin olive oil
- 1 cup chopped parsley
- Freshly ground pepper to taste
- 2 avocados, peeled, pitted, quartered
- 2 red onions, finely chopped
- 1 cup pine nuts, toasted
- 4 teaspoons grated lemon zest
- 6 tablespoons fresh lemon juice
- Sea salt or Himalayan pink salt to

---

[51] Alkaline Recipe: Avocado & Quinoa Salad (Gluten-Free). (2019). Retrieved from https://liveenergized.com/alkaline-recipes/alkaline-quinoa-salad-with-avocado/

taste

- ¼ teaspoon cayenne pepper

Method:

1. Cook the quinoa following the instructions on the package. Transfer into a bowl. Fluff with a fork and set aside for a few minutes to cool slightly.

2. Add rest of the ingredients except avocados and toss well.

1. Divide into plates. Top with avocado pieces and serve.

Kale Caesar Salad[52]

Serves: 3-4

Ingredients:

- 2 very large bunches curly kale, discard the hard stems and ribs, tear the leaves into bite size pieces
- 2/3 cup almonds, chopped
- 1 teaspoon smoked paprika
- 3 teaspoons agave nectar
- 2 cups sunflower seeds + extra for garnishing
- ¼ teaspoon chipotle powder or to taste (optional)
- 4 cloves garlic, minced
- 1 teaspoon sea salt or to taste
- 2 ½ cups water or as required

---

[52] 7 Day Alkaline Diet Plan to Fight Inflammation and Disease With Recipes. (2019). Retrieved from https://www.midlandscbd.com/articles/7-day-alkaline-diet-plan-to-fight-inflammation-and-disease-with-recipes-6882

Method:

2. Place the kale leaves in a large serving bowl.

3. Blend together rest of the ingredients in a blender until smooth.

4. Pour over the kale leaves. Fold gently until the kale leaves are well coated with the dressing.

5. Garnish with sunflower seeds and serve.

Red And White Salad[53]

Serves: 4-6

Ingredients:

- 6 radishes, very thinly sliced
- 1 medium jicama, peeled, quartered, very thinly sliced
- Juice of 2 limes
- ¼ teaspoon salt or to taste
- 2 fennel bulbs, very thinly sliced
- 4 stalks celery, very thinly sliced
- ½ cup avocado oil
- A handful macadamia nuts, chopped, to garnish

Method:

1. Whisk together lemon juice and oil in a large bowl.

---

[53] Red & White Salad of Radish, Fennel, Jicama & Macadamia Nuts– Happy Canada Day! The Alkaline Sisters. (2019). Retrieved from http://www.alkalinesisters.com/red-white-salad-of-radish-fennel-jicama-macadamia-nuts-happy-canada-day/2736/

2. Add rest of the ingredients and toss well.

3. Garnish with macadamia nuts and serve.

pH Balancing Salad54

Serves: 2

Ingredients:

- 10 stalks asparagus, trimmed
- 10 red radishes, thinly sliced
- 1 avocado, peeled, pitted, chopped
- 1 cup chopped alfalfa sprouts
- 1 cup chopped snow pea sprouts
- ½ cup chopped cilantro
- 2 tablespoons pumpkin seeds
- 2 cups chopped arugula
- 2 tablespoons pumpkin seeds, to

54 A Simple pH-Balancing Alkaline Salad. (2019). Retrieved from https://www.mindbodygreen.com/0-14773/a-simple-phbalancing-alkaline-salad.html

garnish

- 1 spring onion, chopped

For dressing:

- 2 teaspoons mustard powder
- 2 tablespoons apple cider vinegar
- Pepper to taste
- 2 tablespoons olive oil
- ½ teaspoon sea salt

Method:

1. Boil asparagus in a saucepan of water (just cover asparagus with water) for 3 minutes or until just tender. Drain and cut into 1 inch pieces diagonally.

2. Add all the ingredients for dressing into a bowl and whisk well.

3. Add all the salad ingredients into the bowl of dressing and toss well.

4. Sprinkle pumpkin seeds on top and serve.

Pomegranate-Carrot-Fennel Salad[55]

Serves: 4

Ingredients:

- 2 pomegranates, peeled, take out the arils
- 10 tablespoons fresh orange juice
- 6 tablespoons fresh lemon juice
- 2 tablespoons extra-virgin olive oil
- 2 fennel bulbs, cut into strips
- 3 cups grated carrot
- Salt to taste
- Pepper to taste
- Pistachio nuts, to garnish

Method:

1. Add orange juice, 3 tablespoons

---

[55] Alkaline Recipes: Pomegranate-Carrot-Fennel Salad. Balance-pH-Diet.com. (2019). Retrieved from https://www.balance-ph-diet.com/alkaline_recipes_pomegranate_salad.html

lemon juice, salt and pepper into a bowl and whisk well.

2. Stir in the pomegranate and carrots.

3. Add fennel, remaining lemon juice, salt and water into another bowl. Whisk well. Set aside for a while.

4. Transfer the fennel mixture into the bowl of pomegranate and toss well.

5. Divide into plates. Top with pistachio nuts and serve.

Raw Green Vegetable Soup56

Serves: 8

Ingredients:

- 2 avocados, peeled, pitted, chopped
- 4 stalks celery, chopped
- 2 small zucchinis, chopped

---

[56] 7 Day Alkaline Diet Plan to Fight Inflammation and Disease With Recipes. (2019). Retrieved from https://www.midlandscbd.com/articles/7-day-alkaline-diet-plan-to-fight-inflammation-and-disease-with-recipes-6882

- 4 cups spinach, torn
- 1 cup chopped cilantro
- ¼ cup chopped onion
- ½ cup chopped parsley
- 4 slices green bell pepper
- ½ cup almonds soaked in water for 4-5 hours
- 3 cups water
- 2 small watermelon radishes, chopped, to garnish
- 2 small cloves garlic, peeled
- Sea salt to taste
- Juice of a lemon or to taste

Method:

1. Add all the ingredients except salt and lemon into a blender and blend until smooth.

2. Pour into a saucepan and place over low heat until just warm. Add salt and

stir. Taste and adjust the seasoning if desired.

3. Add lemon juice and stir.

4. Ladle into soup bowls and serve.

Raw Avocado Broccoli Soup With Cashew Nuts57

Serves: 3-4

Ingredients:

- 1 avocado, peeled, pitted, chopped
- 1 cup cashews
- 2 cloves garlic
- 2 cups broccoli, chopped
- 1 cup alfalfa sprouts
- 1 cup water or alkaline water
- Salt to taste
- Pepper to taste
- 2 tablespoons cold pressed extra-virgin olive oil
- A handful of parsley, chopped, to garnish

Method:

---

57 Free Alkaline Diet Recipes. Balance-pH-Diet.com. (2019). Retrieved from https://www.balance-ph-diet.com/alkaline_recipes.html

1. Add cashews and a little water into a blender and blend until smooth.

2. Add rest of the ingredients except parsley and avocados and blend until smooth.

3. Transfer into a soup pot. Place the pot over low heat until warm.

4. Ladle into soup bowls. Garnish with avocados and parsley and serve.

Super Alkalizing Soup58

Serves: 8

Ingredients:

- 2 teaspoons coconut oil
- 4 cups cubed sweet potato
- 4 celery stalks, chopped
- 12 cups water
- 2 cups parsley, chopped

---

58 Super Alkalising Soup.... (2019). Retrieved from
https://vegiehead.com/blogs/recipes/super-alkalising-soup/

- 1 inch ginger, grated
- 2 tablespoons miso paste
- 2 onions, chopped
- 2 large zucchinis, diced
- 2 cups chopped Roma tomatoes
- 4 cups shredded kale
- 2 cloves garlic, peeled, minced
- 2 teaspoons turmeric powder
- Juice of 2 lemons
- Salt to taste
- 2 teaspoons chia seeds, to garnish
- Steamed greens to serve

Method:

1. Sauté onions in coconut oil in a soup pot until translucent.

2. Add zucchini, sweet potatoes, tomatoes, celery and water and cook until sweet potatoes are tender.

3. Stir in turmeric, ginger, garlic, parsley and kale and cook for a couple of

minutes.

4. Turn off the heat. Cover and set aside for 10 minutes.

5. Stir in miso paste and lemon juice.

6. Ladle into soup bowls. Sprinkle chia seeds on top and serve with steamed greens.

Cream Of Broccoli Soup59

Serves: 8

Ingredients:

- 8 cups water or yeast free broth
- 2 cans (15 ounces each) garbanzo beans drained, rinsed
- 2 onions, chopped
- 2 teaspoons dried thyme
- 3 teaspoons salt

---

59 Alkaline Diet Recipe: Alkaline Cream Of Broccoli Soup. (2019). Retrieved from https://www.getoffyouracid.com/blogs/soups/alkaline-diet-recipe-alkaline-cream-of-broccoli-soup

- ½ teaspoon pepper or to taste
- 8 cups broccoli florets
- 6 cloves garlic, minced or pressed
- 2 sweet potatoes, peeled, chopped into small pieces
- 2 teaspoons celery seeds
- 1 teaspoon dried marjoram or oregano
- ½ teaspoon turmeric powder
- ¼ teaspoon cayenne pepper or to taste

Method:

1. Add all the ingredients into a soup pot and place over medium heat.
2. Cover and cook until tender.
3. Blend with an immersion blender until smooth.
4. Ladle into soup bowls and serve.

Detox Soup Or Broth

[60]Serves: 4

Ingredients:

- 1 cup chopped stalks celery (chopped into chunks)
- 1 cup chopped zucchini (chopped into chunks)
- 1 cup chopped yellow squash, (chopped into chunks)
- 1 cup chopped fresh parsley
- 1 cup green beans, stringed
- 1 cup chopped spinach
- A generous amount of chopped cilantro

<u>Optional:</u>

- 2 cloves garlic, peeled

---

[60] 3 Top Detox Soup Recipes to Promote Alkalinity. (2019). Retrieved from https://universityhealthnews.com/daily/nutrition/3-top-detox-soup-recipes-to-promote-alkalinity/

- 1 onion, chopped
- 2 inch piece ginger, peeled, sliced
- ½ teaspoon turmeric powder
- Cayenne pepper to taste
- 1 teaspoon ground cumin
- 1 tablespoon extra- virgin olive oil

Method:

1. Steam the vegetables until crisp as well as tender. Add onions, ginger and garlic if using, while steaming.

2. Transfer into a blender. Add more water or more if you prefer a soup of thinner consistency.

3. Also add parsley, cilantro spices if using and blend until smooth.

4. Pour the soup back into the pot. Heat the soup thoroughly. Turn off the heat. Add olive oil and stir.

5. Ladle into soup bowls and serve.

Chilled Avocado Tomato Soup61

Serves: 8

Ingredients:

- 4 small avocados, peeled, pitted, chopped
- 2 stalks celery, chopped
- 2 cloves garlic, peeled
- 4 large tomatoes, chopped
- 2 small onions, chopped
- Juice of 2 lemons
- 2 cups water
- A handful parsley, chopped
- Sea salt to taste
- 2 stalks celery, chopped
- 2 cups fresh lovage

Method:

---

61 Alkaline Recipes: Avocado Tomato Soup. Balance-pH-Diet.com. (2019). Retrieved from https://www.balance-ph-diet.com/alkaline_recipes_avocado_tomato_soup.html

1. Add all the ingredients into a blender. Blend until smooth.

2. Pour into a bowl. Cover with cling wrap and chill until use.

Chapter Fifteen: Alkaline Side Dishes

Stir-Fried Greens With Almonds62

Serves: 2

Ingredients:

- 2 small heads broccoli
- 1 small onion, sliced
- 10-12 young beans
- ½ cup chopped cauliflower or

---

62 Alkaline Recipes: Stir-Fried Greens With Almonds. Balance-pH-Diet.com. (2019). Retrieved from https://www.balance-ph-diet.com/alkaline_recipes_stir_fried_greens.html

carrots

- 2 tablespoons cold pressed olive oil
- ¼ teaspoon ground cumin
- ¼ teaspoon dried oregano
- Pepper to taste
- Salt to taste
- 2-3 soaked and sliced almonds, to garnish
- 1 small clove garlic, minced
- 2-3 teaspoons fresh lemon juice

Method:

1. Add all the vegetables in a pan. Place pan over medium heat. Cook until broccoli and beans turn bright green in color. The vegetables should be crisp as well as tender.

2. Stir in the garlic and onion. Sauté for 1-2 minutes. Turn off the heat and transfer into a bowl.

3. To make dressing: Add cumin, oil,

lemon juice, salt, pepper and oregano into a bowl and whisk well.

4. Drizzle over the vegetables in the bowl. Toss lightly.

5. Serve garnished with almond slices.

Vegetable Lasagne[63]

Serves: 4

Ingredients:

- 4 soft avocados, peeled, pitted, chopped
- Juice of 3-4 lemons
- 1 small radish, finely grated
- 2 small leeks, thinly sliced into rings
- 2 red bell peppers, cut into rings
- 2 parsley roots, finely grated
- 2 cloves garlic, peeled
- 2 corn salad greens (also known as lamb's lettuce or field salad greens)
- 2 bunches arugula leaves
- 6 large tomatoes, chopped
- A handful parsley, chopped

---

[63] Alkaline Recipes: Vegetable Lasagne. Balance-pH-Diet.com. (2019). Retrieved from https://www.balance-ph-diet.com/alkaline_recipes_vegetable_lasagne.html

Method:

1. Add avocadoes, garlic and lemon juice into a blender and blend until smooth.

2. Add a little water and blend again.

3. Pour into a bowl. Add radish, parsley root, bell pepper and leeks and stir.

4. To assemble lasagna: Take a casserole dish and spread corn salad greens on the bottom of the dish.

5. Spread avocado mixture evenly.

6. Layer with tomato slices followed by parsley and arugula leaves.

7. Serve.

Mashed Brussels Sprouts With Cauliflower[64]

Serves: 4

Ingredients:

- 4 cups Brussels sprouts
- 1 medium head cauliflower, cut into florets
- 2 cups walnuts
- 1 cup fresh basil
- 1 cup fresh parsley
- 2 cloves garlic, peeled
- 4 tablespoons olive oil
- Sea salt to taste
- Freshly ground pepper to taste
- 1 teaspoon bell pepper powder
- 2 tablespoons lemon juice

---

[64] Alkaline Recipes: Brussels Sprouts with Cauliflower. Balance-pH-Diet.com. (2019). Retrieved from https://www.balance-ph-diet.com/alkaline_recipes_brussels_sprouts.html

Method:

1. Place a saucepan with water over high heat. Add a little salt and bring to a boil.

2. Add cauliflower and cook until soft. Drain and place in a blender.

3. Meanwhile, place another saucepan with water over high heat. Add Brussels sprouts and cook until slightly tender. Drain and place in the blender.

4. Also add walnuts, garlic, bell pepper powder, basil and parsley into the blender and blend until a texture like mashed potatoes is achieved. Add salt and pepper to taste.

5. Add olive oil and lemon juice into a small pan and place the pan over low heat. Whisk well. When the mixture is slightly hot, turn off the heat.

6. Divide cauliflower –Brussels sprout mash among 4 plates. Drizzle olive oil mixture over it and serve.

Mashed Sweet Potatoes65

Serves: 2-3

Ingredients:

- 2 tablespoons cold pressed extra-virgin olive oil
- 3 large sweet potatoes, peeled, cubed
- ¾ -1 cup fresh (preferably) coconut milk
- Salt to taste
- Pepper to taste
- 1 teaspoon curry powder

Method:

---

[65] Alkaline Recipes: Mashed Sweet Potatoes. Balance-pH-Diet.com. (2019). Retrieved from https://www.balance-ph-diet.com/alkaline_recipes_mashed_sweet_potatoes.html

1. Place a pot of water over high heat. Bring to a boil. Add sweet potatoes and cook until soft.

2. Drain and mash with a potato masher, lightly.

3. Add oil, curry powder, coconut milk and mix until well combined. Season with salt and pepper.

4. Serve immediately or heat thoroughly in the microwave just before serving.

Sautéed Zucchini With Toasted Chia Seeds[66]

Serves: 3-4

Ingredients:

- 2 large zucchinis, halved lengthwise, sliced crosswise into semi circles
- 5 tablespoons chia seeds
- 1 teaspoon pepper
- 6 cloves garlic, minced
- 2 teaspoons sea salt
- 2 teaspoons olive oil

Method:

1. Place a skillet over medium-high heat. When the skillet is well heated, add chia seeds and shake the pan often until they become slightly darker in color.

---

[66] Sauteed Zucchini with Toasted Chia Seeds (and health benefits of chia!). Insteading.com (2019). Retrieved from https://insteading.com/blog/chia-seeds-recipe/

Transfer onto a plate and set aside.

2. Lower the heat to medium heat. Add oil, salt, pepper and garlic and stir constantly for a couple of minutes.

3. Stir in the zucchini and raise the heat to medium-high heat. Cook until zucchini is tender. Stir occasionally.

4. Add chia seeds and stir.

5. Serve immediately.

Mediterranean Bell Peppers67

Serves: 4

Ingredients:

- 4 red bell peppers, sliced
- 4 yellow bell peppers, sliced
- 4 cloves garlic, crushed
- 4 medium red onions, thinly sliced
- 4 tablespoons cold pressed extra-

---

[67] Alkaline Recipes: Bell Peppers. Balance-pH-Diet.com. (2019). Retrieved from https://www.balance-ph-diet.com/alkaline_recipes_bell_peppers.html

virgin olive oil

- 2 teaspoons herbes de provence
- ¼ cup chopped fresh parsley
- 2 cups yeast-free vegetable stock
- 2 teaspoons oregano
- Salt to taste
- Pepper to taste

Method:

1. Place a pan over medium heat. Add oil and heat. Add onion and bell peppers and sauté until slightly tender.

2. Add garlic and sauté until aromatic.

3. Stir in the stock, salt, pepper, parsley and herbes de provence

4. Cover and cook until tender.

5. Serve hot.

Grilled Veggies68

---

[68] Alkaline Recipes: Grilled Veggies. Balance-pH-Diet.com. (2019). Retrieved from https://www.balance-ph-diet.com/alkaline_recipes_grilled_veggies.html

Serves: 2

Ingredients:

- 1 medium eggplant, chopped into chunks
- 1 medium zucchini, chopped into chunks
- ½ yellow bell pepper, chopped into 1 inch squares
- ½ red bell pepper, chopped into 1 inch squares
- ½ green bell pepper, chopped into 1 inch squares
- 1 medium onion, chopped into 1 inch squares, separate the layers
- 1 clove garlic, peeled
- 2 carrots, sliced
- 1 ½ tablespoons cold pressed extra-virgin olive oil
- Sea salt to taste
- Freshly ground pepper to taste

- Fresh herbs of your choice, minced

Method:

1. Place all the vegetables in a baking dish. Season with salt and pepper. Drizzle oil over it. Sprinkle herbs. Toss well. Spread it evenly.

2. Grill in a preheated oven at 325 ° F for about 20-30 minutes. Stir a couple of times while grilling.

3. Serve hot.

Alkaline Fried Rice69

Serves: 4

Ingredients:

- 2 cups wild rice
- 4 cups water

---

69 Alkaline Electric Fried Rice - Ty's Conscious Kitchen. (2019). Retrieved from https://www.tysconsciouskitchen.com/dr-sebi-alkaline-electric-fried-rice/

- ½ cup diced butternut squash
- ½ cup diced green onions
- ½ cup diced white onions
- ½ cup diced green bell pepper
- ½ cup red bell pepper
- 2 teaspoons minced ginger
- 1 teaspoon onion powder
- 1 teaspoon basil
- 1 teaspoon sea salt
- Grape seed oil, as required
- ½ teaspoon crushed red pepper
- 1 teaspoon sesame seeds (optional)
- 1 cup scrambled egg

Method:

1. Pour broth and water into a pot. Add rice. Place pot over high heat.

2. Cover and let it come to a boil.

3. Lower the heat to medium heat and cook until dry. Stir occasionally. Turn off the heat. Fluff with a fork.

4. Place a large skillet or wok over medium heat. Add 3-4 tablespoons grapeseed oil. When the oil is heated, add all the vegetables, salt, pepper and crushed red pepper and sauté until tender.

5. Stir in the scrambled eggs, wild rice and sesame seeds. Stir fry for 4-5 minutes.

6. Serve with some alkaline curry or gravy.

Alkaline Macaroni And Cheese70

Serves: 4-5

Ingredients:

- 6 ounces kamut spirals or any other alkaline pasta of your choice
- 2 tablespoons garbanzo flour (chickpea flour)
- 1 teaspoon grape seed oil
- ½ teaspoon sea salt
- 1 tablespoon lime juice
- ¼ pound raw brazil nuts, soaked overnight
- ½ cup spring water
- 1 teaspoon onion powder
- ¼ teaspoon ground annatto
- 2 cups hemp milk or coconut milk

---

[70] Alkaline Electric Macaroni and Cheese - Ty's Conscious Kitchen. (2019). Retrieved from https://www.tysconsciouskitchen.com/dr-sebi-alkaline-electric-macaroni-and-cheese/

Method:

1. Cook the pasta following the directions on the package. Set aside.

2. Add rest of the ingredients into a blender and blend until smooth.

3. Pour into a greased baking dish. Add pasta and stir.

4. Bake in a preheated oven at 325°F for about 20-30 minutes. Broil for a few minutes if you want a crisp top.

Lentils And Amaranth Patties[71]

Serves: 7-8

Ingredients:

- ¼ cup amaranth
- ½ cup red lentils
- 1 small onion, chopped

---

[71] Protein Power Amaranth Patties. (2019). Gourmandelle.com. Retrieved from https://gourmandelle.com/amaranth-patties-chiftelute-de-amaranth/

- ¼ cup chopped parsley
- 1 tablespoon psyllium husks
- ¼ cup whole wheat or gluten-free breadcrumbs
- Salt to taste
- Pepper to taste
- 2 tablespoons nutritional yeast
- Few black olives, pitted, sliced (optional but suggested)
- Oil, to fry, as required

Method:

1. Place amaranth and lentils in a saucepan. Pour enough water to cover.

2. Place over medium heat and cook until tender.

3. Drain and place in a bowl. Add rest of the ingredients except oil and mix well. If the mixture is too moist, add some more bread crumbs.

4. Divide the mixture into 7-8 equal

portions and shape into patties.

5. Place a nonstick pan over medium heat. Add a little oil and heat. Fry the patties in batches until golden brown on both the sides.

6. Remove with a slotted spoon and place on a plate lined with paper towels.

7. Serve hot with a dip of your choice.

Chapter Sixteen: Alkaline Meals

Californian Avocado Toasts[72]

Serves: 2

Ingredients:

- 4 slices whole wheat bread, toasted
- 2 tablespoons salted cashews
- 1 teaspoon chia seeds
- ½ Californian avocado, peeled, pitted, sliced
- 2 tablespoons craisins

Method:

1. Place avocado slices over the bread slices. Sprinkle craisins and chia seeds. Place cashews over it and serve.

---

[72] California Avocado Toasts - 4 Ways. (2019). Retrieved from
https://iwashyoudry.com/california-avocado-toasts/

Purple Pasta With Walnut Pesto And Tender Stem Broccoli[73]

Serves: 4-5

Ingredients:

For the broccoli:

- 2 packs tender stem broccoli
- Salt to taste
- 1 cup tamari
- 1 cup olive oil

For the pasta:

- 12 courgettes
- 4 cups grated beetroot
- Salt to taste
- ½ cup olive oil

---

[73] Rodgers, A. (2015). Recipe: Purple Pasta With Walnut Pesto & Tenderstem Broccoli. Retrieved from https://www.collective-evolution.com/2015/08/26/recipe-purple-pasta-with-walnut-pesto-tenderstem-broccoli/

For the walnut pesto:

- 4 cups basil
- 2 cups walnuts
- ½ cup olive oil
- Salt to taste
- 4 tablespoons lemon juice

Method:

2. To make the broccoli: Remove the broccoli florets and cut into smaller florets and place in a large bowl. Add rest of the ingredients and set aside to marinate for at least 2 hours. Drain.

3. To make the pasta: Using a mandolin slicer, slice the courgette. Make small stacks of the courgette and then cut it into strips such that it resembles linguine pasta strips.

4. Place beetroots in a large bowl. Add the courgette strips and mix well. Add rest of the ingredients and set aside for a

few hours until it turns purple. Then place in a strainer or colander for a while to drain off the liquid.

5. To make walnut pesto: Add all the ingredients for walnut pesto into a food processor and pulse until a chunky consistency is achieved.

6. To assemble: Mix together the purple pasta and pesto in a bowl. Place the broccoli on a serving platter. Place the purple pasta over it and serve.

Mexican Quinoa74

Serves: 2-3

Ingredients:

- ½ cup fresh or frozen corn kernels
- ½ cup quinoa, rinsed
- ½ cup salsa
- ½ cup vegetable broth
- ½ can (from a 15 ounces can) black beans, drained
- ½ tablespoon ground cumin
- ½ teaspoon chili powder
- ½ tablespoon olive oil
- 1 jalapeño, minced
- Salt to taste
- Pepper to taste
- A handful pumpkin seeds, to garnish
- A handful cilantro, chopped, to garnish

---

[74] 5-ingredient Mexican Quinoa. Simply Quinoa.com (2019). Retrieved from https://www.simplyquinoa.com/5-ingredient-mexican-quinoa/

- Lime juice to taste

Method:

1. Place a skillet over medium high heat. Add oil and heat. Stir in jalapeño and garlic and sauté for a minute.

2. Add quinoa, broth, beans, chili powder, salsa, salt, pepper and cumin and stir.

3. When it begins to boil, lower the heat and cover with a lid. Cook until dry.

4. Add lime juice and cilantro and stir.

5. Sprinkle pumpkin seeds on top and serve.

Easy Green Casserole75

Serves: 2-3

Ingredients:

- 1 ½ cups chopped kale, packed
- 1 cup chopped broccoli
- 1 ½ cups cooked quinoa
- ¼ cup chopped onion

For sauce:

- 1 cup full fat coconut milk
- 2 tablespoons nutritional yeast
- ½ teaspoon sea salt
- ¼ teaspoon rosemary
- ½ can (cannellini beans), drained
- ½ teaspoon pepper
- ¼ teaspoon dried thyme
- ¼ teaspoon cayenne pepper

[75] Easy Green Casserole [Vegan]. (2019). Retrieved from
https://www.onegreenplanet.org/vegan-recipe/easy-green-casserole/

Method:

1. Add all the ingredients for sauce into a blender and blend until smooth.

2. Add kale, broccoli, quinoa and onion into a baking dish and stir. Pour the blended sauce all over the mixture.

3. Bake in a preheated oven at 375ºF until golden brown at a few spots on top.

4. Cool slightly and serve.

Millet Stir Fry With Vegetables[76]

Serves: 4

Ingredients:

- 2 cups little millet or proso millet cheena millet
- 2 inches ginger, peeled, grated
- 2 onions, chopped
- 4 cloves garlic, minced
- 1 ½ teaspoons ground turmeric
- 2 teaspoons ground coriander
- Red pepper flakes, to taste
- 4 teaspoons ground cumin
- Salt to taste
- 2 tablespoons vegetable oil
- 4 cloves garlic, minced
- 2 green chilies, halved lengthwise, deseeded
- 2 cups chopped mixed vegetables of

[76] Millet stir fry with vegetables. My Weekend Kitchen. (2019). Retrieved from https://www.myweekendkitchen.in/millet-stir-fry-vegetables/

your choice

- 4 cups water or vegetable broth
- A handful fresh cilantro, chopped to garnish
- A handful toasted almonds, chopped

Method:

1. Place millet on a fine wire mesh strainer. Rinse under running water. Place in a bowl and cover with water. Set aside for 10-15 minutes. Drain and set aside.

2. Place a large skillet or pot over medium heat. Add oil and heat. Add ginger, garlic and green chili and stir for 40-60 seconds or until aromatic.

3. Stir in the onion, spices and mixed vegetables. Cook for a couple of minutes.

4. Add millet, salt and broth and stir. Bring to a boil.

5. Lower the heat and cover partially.

Cook until dry.

    6. Sprinkle cilantro and almonds on top and serve.

Burrito Bowl77

Serves: 4

Ingredients:

- 2 cups brown rice, rinsed, cook the rice according to the instructions on the package
- 8 green onions, thinly sliced
- 8 cloves garlic, minced
- Juice of 2 limes or to taste
- 4 avocado, peeled, pitted sliced
- 4 cans (15 ounces each) adzuki beans
- 1 teaspoon ground cumin

---

[77] Alkaline Diet Recipe: Burrito Bowl. (2019). Retrieved from https://www.getoffyouracid.com/blogs/main-course/alkaline-diet-recipe-burrito-bowl

- A handful fresh cilantro, chopped
- Salt to taste
- 2 tablespoons toasted sesame seeds
- Hot sauce, to drizzle

Method:

1. Place a skillet over low heat. Add garlic, cumin, salt, black beans, green onions and stir. Let it simmer for around 10 minutes.

2. Divide the rice into individual serving bowls. Serve the bean mixture over it.

3. Top with avocados, sesame seeds and cilantro and serve.

Wild Rice With Alkalizing Greens[78]

Serves: 8

Ingredients:

- 2 cups wild rice, rinsed
- 2 cups finely chopped broccoli florets
- 4 carrots, finely chopped
- 2 cups yeast-free vegetable broth or water + extra to steam fry
- 2 cups finely chopped Pak Choi
- 4 stalks celery, finely chopped
- 2 cups finely chopped bean sprouts
- 2 cups young beans
- 2 chilies, finely chopped
- A handful fresh cilantro, chopped
- A handful fresh basil, chopped

---

[78] Alkaline Recipes: Wild Rice. Balance-pH-Diet.com. (2019). Retrieved from https://www.balance-ph-diet.com/alkaline_recipes_wild_rice_greens.html

Method:

1. Add broth and wild rice into a pot and stir. Place over medium heat. When it begins to boil, lower the heat and cover with a lid. Cook until tender.

2. Uncover and fluff with a fork. Let it rest for 10 minutes.

3. Meanwhile, place a skillet over medium heat. Add all the vegetables and 1-2 tablespoons broth and sauté until vegetables are crisp as well as tender.

4. Place chili and cilantro in a mortar and pound with a pestle until a paste is formed. Add lime juice and stir.

5. Divide wild rice among individual serving plates. Divide the vegetable mixture and place over the rice.

6. Garnish with basil and serve.

Super Seeds Pancakes79

Serves: 6

Ingredients:

- ½ cup pumpkin seeds
- ½ cup flax seeds
- 2 cups buckwheat groats
- ½ cup sesame seeds
- ½ cup chia seeds
- 2 teaspoons baking soda
- 1 teaspoon baking powder
- ½ cup nondairy milk of your choice or more if required
- 1 teaspoon stevia extract
- 2 teaspoons coconut oil

Method:

1. Grind together all the seeds and buckwheat groats until fine in texture.

---

[79] Marks, E. (2019). 12 Easy and Delicious Alkaline Breakfast Recipes For Energy. Retrieved from https://great4you.co/alkaline-breakfast-recipes/

2. Transfer into a mixing bowl.

3. Add rest of the ingredients except coconut oil into the mixing bowl and stir. Add more milk if the batter is very thick. Let the batter sit for 10 minutes.

4. Place a nonstick pan over medium heat.

5. Add ½ teaspoon oil and swirl the pan so spread the oil. When the pan is well heated, pour ¼ cup batter on the pan and swirl the pan so that the batter is thinly spread.

6. In a while bubbles will appear on the top of the pancakes. Flip sides when the underside is golden brown and cook the other side. Remove from the pan and keep warm.

7. Repeat steps 5-6 and make remaining pancakes. Use more oil if required.

8. Serve with maple syrup if desired.

Cauliflower Cheese-Stuffed Sweet Potatoes80

Serves: 8

Ingredients:

- 8 sweet potatoes
- 1 cup nutritional yeast
- 1 head cauliflower, cut into florets
- 1 cup vegetable broth or water
- 1 teaspoon cayenne pepper
- 2 tablespoons white miso
- 2 teaspoons tahini
- 2 tablespoons balsamic vinegar
- 8 sundried tomatoes
- 40 fresh basil leaves
- 2 garlic cloves, peeled
- 2 small chili peppers
- 2 tablespoons lemon juice

---

80 Cauliflower Cheese-Stuffed Sweet Potatoes [Vegan]. (2019). Retrieved from https://www.onegreenplanet.org/vegan-recipe/cauliflower-cheese-stuffed-sweet-potatoes/

- 1 ½ cups diced tempeh
- 2 tablespoons apple cider vinegar
- 2 cups chopped kale, discard hard stems and ribs
- 2/3 cup pecans

Method:

1. For sweet potatoes: Prick the sweet potatoes at a few places and place on a baking sheet.

2. Roast in a preheated oven at 360 º F until cooked through.

3. Place a large pot of water over medium heat. Bring to a boil. Add cauliflower and cook until soft. Drain and set aside to cool for a few minutes.

4. Meanwhile make the cheese sauce as follows: Add cauliflower, broth, cayenne pepper, miso, tahini, nutritional yeast, garlic, chili and lemon juice into a blender and blend until creamy.

5. Place a skillet over medium heat. Add both the vinegars and tempeh and stir until well coated.

6. Place over high heat and cook until slightly crisp.

7. Split the sweet potatoes. Press the ends slightly. Fill the sweet potatoes with the cheese sauce. Place kale, sun dried tomatoes and pecans on top and serve.

Spiced Coconut Dal[81]

Serves: 2-3

Ingredients:

- ½ tablespoon coconut oil
- ½ teaspoon mustard seeds
- 1 small yellow onion, chopped
- A pinch chipotle chili powder
- ½ teaspoon ground cumin
- ½ teaspoon sea salt
- ¾ cup split red lentils
- 1 ½ cups water
- 2 bay leaves
- ½ teaspoon cumin seeds
- ¼ teaspoon fenugreek seeds
- A pinch cayenne pepper
- ½ teaspoon ground coriander
- ¼ teaspoon ground turmeric
- Freshly ground pepper to taste

---

[81] Spiced Coconut Dal [Vegan]. (2019). Retrieved from
https://www.onegreenplanet.org/vegan-recipe/spiced-coconut-dal/

- 1 small Roma tomato, diced
- 1 cup full fat coconut milk

For optional toppings:

- Tempeh, cubed
- Sautéed onion
- Greens

Method:

1. Place a saucepan over medium heat. Add oil and heat. When the oil is heated, add mustard, cumin and fenugreek. When they splutter, add onion and sauté until translucent.
2. Add all the spices and salt and stir.
3. Stir in lentils, water and tomatoes.
4. When the mixture begins to boil, lower the heat and cover with a lid. Simmer until lentils are slightly tender.
5. Add bay leaves and coconut milk and simmer until lentils are tender.

6. Cool for a few minutes and serve topped with optional toppings if using.

Roasted Spiced Carrots82

Serves: 4-8

Ingredients:

<u>For spiced carrots:</u>

- 3 pounds carrots, peeled
- 2 teaspoons cumin seeds, toasted, ground
- 2 teaspoons paprika
- 2 teaspoons fennel seeds, toasted, ground
- 2 tablespoons sunflower oil
- ½ teaspoon salt

<u>For tahini sauce:</u>

- 2 small cloves garlic, peeled
- juice of a lemon
- water, as required

---

82 Roasted Spiced Carrots [Vegan]. (2019). Retrieved from https://www.onegreenplanet.org/vegan-recipe/roasted-spiced-carrots/

- ½ cup tahini
- ½ teaspoon salt

For assembling:

- ½ cup toasted pumpkin seeds
- 2 cups cooked wild rice
- ½ cup toasted pine nuts
- alfalfa sprouts

Method:

1. For spiced carrots: Place a sheet of parchment paper on a large baking sheet.

2. Place carrots in a large bowl. Mix together all the spices and salt in a bowl and sprinkle over the carrots. Toss well.

3. Drizzle oil over the carrots. Toss well.

4. Spread the carrots in a single layer, on the prepared baking sheet. Use 2 baking sheets if required.

5. Bake in a preheated oven at 300° F

for about 20-25 minutes or until carrots are tender inside and firm outside. Stir once halfway through baking.

6. For tahini sauce:__Add all the ingredients for tahini sauce into a blender and blend until smooth. Pour into a bowl.

7. To assemble: Divide the wild rice into bowls. Layer with carrots. Sprinkle pumpkin seeds, pine nuts and alfalfa sprouts on top and serve.

Alkaline Root Curry83

Serves: 6-8

Ingredients:

- 2 large carrots, peeled, cubed
- 2 beetroots, peeled, cubed
- 2 parsnips, peeled, cubed

---

[83] Alkaline Diet Recipe #110: Alkaline Root Vegetable Curry. (2019). Live Energized.com. Retrieved from https://liveenergized.com/alkaline-recipes/alkaline-diet-recipe-110-alkaline-root-vegetable-curry/

- 2 celeriac, peeled, cubed
- 6 cloves garlic, chopped
- 4 tablespoons grape seed oil or rapeseed oil
- 4 large onions, chopped
- 2 red chili peppers, chopped
- 2 cans (14.1 ounces each) chopped tomatoes, chopped
- 1 teaspoon ground turmeric
- 4 sticks cinnamon
- 3 teaspoons cumin seeds
- 2 teaspoons fennel seeds
- 2 cups coconut milk
- ½ cup fresh cilantro, chopped
- 4 teaspoons coriander seeds
- 2 inches fresh ginger, peeled, sliced
- Juice of 2 limes
- Salt to taste
- Pepper to taste

Method:

1. Place the root vegetables on a baking sheet. Sprinkle about 2 tablespoons oil over it. Toss well. Spread it evenly. Use 2 baking sheets if required.

2. Bake in a preheated oven at 350° F for about 20-25 minutes or until soft.

3. Meanwhile, place a heavy bottomed skillet over medium heat. Add cumin, coriander and fennel seeds and roast until fragrant. Remove from the pan and pound into a rough powder.

4. Add onions, garlic, ginger and chili into a blender and blend until smooth.

5. Place the skillet back on heat. Add remaining oil. When the oil is heated, add cinnamon and onion paste and sauté until light brown. Add tomatoes and cook for 3-4 minutes.

6. Add turmeric and the powder mixture and sauté for a couple of minutes.

7. Add coconut milk and the roasted root vegetables. Heat thoroughly.

8. Serve over cooked brown rice or cauliflower rice.

Chapter Seventeen: Alkaline Teas

Ginger & Turmeric Refresher Tea84

Serves: 1

Ingredients:

- 1 ¼ cups filtered water, preferably alkaline water
- ½ inch minced or grated fresh turmeric
- ½ inch minced or grated ginger
- A pinch black pepper (optional)

Method:

1. Add all the ingredients into a

84 Two Powerful Anti-Inflammatory Turmeric & Ginger Teas (Free Alkaline Recipes #172 & #173!). (2019). Live Energized.com. Retrieved from https://liveenergized.com/alkaline-recipes/two-powerful-anti-inflammatory-turmeric-ginger-teas/

saucepan. Place saucepan over medium heat and bring to a boil.

2. Lower the heat and simmer for 5-6 minutes or for longer if you want stronger tea.

3. Strain and serve hot or chilled.

Ojito Fat Flush Water85

Serves: 2

Ingredients:

- 1 lime, sliced
- 3-4 thin lemon sliced
- Water, as required to fill
- 1 small cucumber, thinly sliced
- 10 fresh mint leaves, torn

Method:

---

[85] Mojito Fat Flush Water & Detox Dream Water. (2019). Retrieved from https://www.getoffyouracid.com/blogs/alkaline-recipes/mojito-fat-flush-water-detox-dream-water

1. Add all the ingredients into a jug. Cover and chill overnight.

2. Pour into glasses and serve.

Fennel and Mint Tea[86]

Serves: 2-3

Ingredients:

- 2 teabags fennel tea
- ½ cup fresh mint leaves
- 4 inches fresh ginger, peeled, sliced
- 4 cups alkaline water

Method:

1. Pour water into a saucepan. Place saucepan over medium heat and bring to a boil.

2. Add ginger and boil for 6-7 minutes. Remove from heat.

3. Drop the teabags and mint leaves in the water. Cover and let it steep for 10 minutes.

---

[86] Tuchowska, M. (2019). Warm-Up Alkaline Drinks - Holistic Wellness Project. Retrieved from https://www.holisticwellnessproject.com/blog/alkaline-diet/warm-alkaline-drinks/

4. Strain and pour into cups.

5. Serve immediately.

Rooibos And Almond Milk Drink[87]

Serves: 2-3

Ingredients:

- 4 bags rooibos tea
- 1 cup almond milk
- 4 cups alkaline water
- 1 inch ginger, peeled, sliced

Method:

1. Pour water into a saucepan. Place saucepan over medium heat and bring to a boil. Remove from heat.

2. Drop the teabags and ginger in the water. Cover and let it steep for 5

[87] Tuchowska, M. (2019). Warm-Up Alkaline Drinks - Holistic Wellness Project. Retrieved from https://www.holisticwellnessproject.com/blog/alkaline-diet/warm-alkaline-drinks/

minutes.

3. Strain and divide into cups. Divide almond milk into the cups and stir.

4. Serve immediately.

Lemon Balm Tea88

Serves: 2

Ingredients:

- 2 cups water, boiling hot
- 4 teaspoons finely chopped fresh lemon balm leaves

Method:

1. Add all the ingredients into a teapot. Cover and let it steep for 10 minutes.

2. Strain and pour into cups.

3. Serve immediately.

---

88 Lemon Balm Tea - A Soothing and Healing Tea. (2019). Retrieved from https://www.therighttea.com/lemon-balm-tea.html

Chamomile Tea89

Serves: 2

Ingredients:

- 2 handfuls fresh chamomile flowers
- 4 apple mint leaves (optional)
- 2 cups boiling hot spring water

Method:

1. Pour boiling hot water into a teapot. Place chamomile flowers and mint leaves in a cheese cloth or infuser and drop into the teapot. Cover the lid of the teapot. Let it steep for 5 minutes.

2. Discard the mint leaves and chamomile flowers and serve.

Lavender And Chamomile Tea90

---

89 How to Make Chamomile Tea: 5 Recipes From Simple Tea to a Hot Toddy - Cup & Leaf. (2019). Retrieved from https://www.cupandleaf.com/blog/how-to-make-chamomile-tea

Serves: 2-3

Ingredients:

- ¼ cup fresh lavender flowers
- ¼ cup fresh chamomile flowers
- ¼ cup fresh apple mint leaves
- Sweetener to taste
- Juice of a lemon
- 4 cups hot water

Method:

1. Pour hot water into a teapot. Place lavender flowers, chamomile flowers and mint leaves in the teapot. Cover the lid of the teapot. Let it steep for 5 minutes.

2. Strain and add lemon juice and sweetener and stir.

3. Pour into cups and serve.

---

[90] How to Make Chamomile Tea: 5 Recipes From Simple Tea to a Hot Toddy. (2019). Cup & Leaf. Retrieved from
https://www.cupandleaf.com/blog/how-to-make-chamomile-tea

Iced Peppermint Tea91

Serves: 2

Ingredients:

- handful of fresh peppermint leaves or 2 teaspoons dried mint leaves 2 peppermint tea bags
- juice of a lime or lemon
- 2 cups hot water
- sweetener to taste

Method:

1. If using fresh peppermint leaves, slightly crush the leaves.

2. Pour hot water into a teapot. Add peppermint leaves and cover. Let it steep for 10 minutes.

3. Strain and add lemon juice and an

---

91 How to Make Peppermint Tea 5 Different Ways. (2019). Cup & Leaf. Retrieved from https://www.cupandleaf.com/blog/how-to-make-peppermint-tea

alkaline-friendly sweetener, if desired.

4. Chill and serve with crushed ice.

Fruit-Infused Peppermint Tea92

Serves: 4

Ingredients:

- 1 cup loosely packed fresh mint leaves, slightly crushed.
- ¾ cup fruit of your choice like berries, figs, apricot, cherries, citrus fruits etc.
- 4 cups boiling hot water
- sweetener to taste

Method:

1. Pour hot water into a teapot. Add peppermint leaves and cover. Let it steep

---

92 How to Make Peppermint Tea 5 Different Ways. (2019). Cup & Leaf. Retrieved from https://www.cupandleaf.com/blog/how-to-make-peppermint-tea

for 10 minutes.

2. Strain and add sweetener. Pour into a jug. Add the fruit that you prefer.

3. Chill and serve with crushed ice.

Chapter Eighteen: Alkaline Desserts

Strawberry Coconut Chia Pudding93

Serves: 4

Ingredients:

- 6 tablespoons chia seeds
- 2 tablespoons agave nectar
- 4 cups fresh strawberries, retain a few to garnish
- 2 cups coconut milk
- 2 teaspoons pure vanilla extract
- 2 tablespoons coconut flakes

---

93 Strawberry Chia Pudding. (2019). Retrieved from https://www.pcrm.org/good-nutrition/plant-based-diets/recipes/strawberry-chia-pudding

Method:

1. Add chia seeds and coconut milk into a bowl and mix well.

2. Stir in vanilla and agave and cover the bowl with cling wrap. Chill for 4-5 hours.

3. Blend strawberries in a blender until smooth. Pour into the bowl of chia seeds and stir.

4. Divide into dessert bowls or glasses.

5. Garnish with coconut flakes and strawberries and serve.

Raw Pumpkin Pie94

Serves: 10-15

Ingredients:

For pie crust:

- 2 cups raw almonds
- 2 cups pitted dates or Turkish apricots
- 2 cups unsweetened coconut flakes
- 2 teaspoons ground cinnamon

For pie filling:

- 2 cups pecans, soaked in water overnight
- 12 dates, pitted
- 1 teaspoon ground nutmeg
- 2 ½ cups pumpkin puree

---

94 Alkaline Diet Recipe: Raw Pumpkin Pie. (2019). Retrieved from https://www.getoffyouracid.com/blogs/desserts/alkaline-diet-recipe-raw-pumpkin-pie

- 1 teaspoon ground cinnamon + extra to garnish
  - 2 teaspoons pure vanilla extract
  - ½ teaspoon sea salt
  - 2 teaspoons tamari (optional)

Method:

1. To make crust: Add all the ingredients for crust into the food processor bowl. Process until oil is visible and the mixture sticks together.

2. Divide the mixture into 2 tart pans or pie pans. Press the mixture on to the bottom as well as the sides of the pans.

3. To make filling: Add all the ingredients for filling into a blender and blend until smooth.

4. Spoon the mixture on the crust. Spread it evenly. Garnish with ground cinnamon.

5. Chill for a few hours.

6. Remove from the mold. Cut into wedges and serve.

Ginger Cinnamon Fruit With Sweet Tahini Dip95

Serves: 4

Ingredients:

For ginger cinnamon fruit:

- 2 apples, peeled, cored, chopped into bite size cubes
- 2 pears, chopped into bite size cubes
- 2 teaspoons sea salt
- 4-6 tablespoons fresh ginger, peeled, finely grated
- 2 teaspoons ground cinnamon

For sweet tahini dip:

- 6 tablespoons raw almond butter

---

95 Alkaline Diet Recipe: Ginger Cinnamon Fruit with Sweet Tahini Dip. (2019). Retrieved from
https://www.getoffyouracid.com/blogs/desserts/18889199-alkaline-diet-recipe-ginger-cinnamon-fruit-with-sweet-tahini-dip

- 6 tablespoons tahini
- 2 tablespoons coconut nectar or honey
- 4 teaspoons tamari
- 4 tablespoons coconut oil
- ½ teaspoon cayenne pepper

Method:

1. To make ginger cinnamon fruit: Add ginger, salt and cinnamon into a bowl and stir.

2. Add fruits and stir. Chill until use.

3. To make sweet tahini dip: Add almond butter, tahini, coconut nectar, tamari, coconut oil and cayenne pepper into a bowl and whisk until well combined.

4. Divide the fruits into dessert bowls. Drizzle sweet tahini dip on top and serve.

Chocolate Banana Fro-Yo96

Serves: 4

Ingredients:

- 4 bananas, sliced, frozen
- 2 -3 tablespoons raw almond butter
- 6 tablespoons raw cacao powder
- ¼- ½ cup unsweetened almond milk
- 2 tablespoons hemp seeds, to garnish
- 2 tablespoons chia seeds, to garnish
- Ground cinnamon, to garnish

Method:

1. Add cacao and bananas into a blender and blend until well combined.

2. Add ¼ cup almond milk, chia seeds and hemp seeds and blend until just combined. Add more almond milk if

---

[96] Coco Banana Fro-Yo. (2019). Retrieved from
https://www.getoffyouracid.com/blogs/desserts/coco-banana-fro-yo

desired.

3. Pour into dessert bowls. Garnish with hemp seeds and chia seeds and serve.

Strawberry Mango Frozen Fruit Bars97

Serves: 6-8

Ingredients:

- 1 ½ cups frozen strawberries
- 2/3 cup water, divided
- ½ cup frozen chopped mango
- 1 teaspoon powdered stevia, divided

Method:

1. Add strawberries. ½ teaspoon stevia and 1/3 cup water into a blender and

97 Amazing Raw Vegan Dessert Recipes - Holistic Wellness Project. (2019). Retrieved from https://www.holisticwellnessproject.com/blog/alkaline-diet/raw-vegan-dessert-recipes/

blend until smooth.

2. Divide into 6-8 popsicle molds.

3. Clean the blender.

4. Add mango, ½ teaspoon stevia and 1/3 cup water into the blender and blend until smooth.

5. Pour over the strawberry layer in the molds.

6. Insert popsicle sticks into the molds. Freeze until firm.

7. Remove from the mold and serve.

Sweet & Easy Strawberry Sorbet98

Serves: 8-10

Ingredients:

- 5 cups sliced fresh strawberries

---

98 Amazing Raw Vegan Dessert Recipes - Holistic Wellness Project. (2019). Retrieved from https://www.holisticwellnessproject.com/blog/alkaline-diet/raw-vegan-dessert-recipes/

- 8-10 drops stevia
- 1 ½ cups thick coconut milk

Method:

1. Add strawberries and coconut milk into a blender and blend until. Add stevia and blend again.

2. Serve right away or freeze until slightly firm and serve.

Frozen Chocolate Tropical Monkey[99]

Serves: 4

Ingredients:

- 4 frozen bananas
- 4 tablespoons cacao powder
- 4 tablespoons chia seeds

[99] Alkaline Diet Recipe: Frozen Chocolate Tropical Monkey. (2019). Retrieved from https://www.getoffyouracid.com/blogs/desserts/alkaline-diet-recipe-frozen-chocolate-tropical-monkey

- 4 tablespoons coconut oil
- 2 tablespoons cacao nibs
- 4 cups coconut milk

Method:

1. Add all the ingredients except chia seeds into a blender and blend until smooth.

2. Add chia seeds and pulse for 4-5 seconds.

3. Pour into dessert bowls.

4. Serve immediately.

Conclusion

As you come to the end of this book, I would like to thank you for investing your time and money on it. I hope you found it resourceful and that it was a good read.

By now, you should have a good grasp on how to proceed with switching from an unhealthy diet to the alkaline diet. It is an extremely effective and healthy diet that many others have tried and found to be beneficial. This diet will help you improve your overall health and well-being. Choosing to go on this path is not something you will regret. Try not to expect instantaneous results and stick with the diet for a while to see its work in action. If you go about it the right way, anyone can benefit from this diet.

Follow the guidelines given in this book to help you as you begin the alkaline diet. The sample diet plan will be a good way to get started. Also, you can make use of the many recipes we have curated here for you to try. These delicious alkaline-friendly recipes will make your meals much better and the diet much easier to follow through with.

If you find this book useful and see good results from following the alkaline diet, you can even recommend it to family or friends who might find it useful. Nonetheless, I assure you that this diet will help you see results that will make the effort worthwhile.

References

The Alkaline Diet: An Evidence-Based Review. (2019). Retrieved from https://www.healthline.com/nutrition/the-alkaline-diet-myth

Katherine Marengo LDN, R. (2019). Alkaline diet: Claims, facts, and foods. Retrieved from https://www.medicalnewstoday.com/articles/324271.php

Brown, D. (2019). Alkaline For Life Diet Plan— Better Bones. Retrieved from https://www.betterbones.com/alkaline-balance/diet-plan/

Top 10 Alkaline Foods You Should Be Eating Everyday. (2019). Retrieved from https://www.youtube.com/watch?v=qu645wvzMwQ

Alkaline Diet Plan Review: Does It Work?

(2019). Retrieved from
https://www.webmd.com/diet/a-z/alkaline-
diets

Is an Alkaline Diet the Key to Longevity?
(2019). Retrieved from
https://draxe.com/alkaline-diet/

Brown, D. (2019). Alkaline Forming Foods
List— Better Bones. Retrieved from
https://www.betterbones.com/alkaline-
balance/alkaline-forming-foods/

Alkaline Diet Plan. Livestrong.com. (2019).
Retrieved from
https://www.livestrong.com/article/221991-
alkaline-diet-plan/

Free Complete Alkaline Food Chart. (2019).
Retrieved from
https://www.avocadoninja.co.uk/pages/free-
alkaline-food-chart

www.ingramcontent.com/pod-product-compliance
Lightning Source LLC
Chambersburg PA
CBHW062130280526
45788CB00001B/114